Beyond Breath

Beyond Breath

Monis

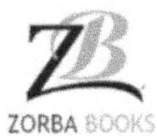

ZORBA BOOKS

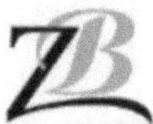

ZORBA BOOKS

Publishing Services in India by Zorba Books, 2018

Website: www.zorbabooks.com
Email: info@zorbabooks.com

Copyright © MANISH SHAH, 2018

Print Book ISBN: 978-93-87456-89-1
eBook ISBN: 978-93-87456-90-7

Zorba Books Pvt. Ltd.(opc)
Gurgaon, INDIA

Printed at Repro Knowledgecast Limited, Thane

This book is dedicated to my mother.

Preface

This book is about Bio-hacking.

The dictionary may give a different definition of the word, but my understanding of this term is very different.

All my life, I have observed people chasing money and material goals throughout their lives. When they begin to realize these transient goals, the realization slowing starts sinking in that 'spending more time on this beautiful planet' is more important than having more money in the bank. And the sad trade-off is that they end up-spending all their hard-earned money on their lost health.

This book is my attempt to dig into that aspect of our tragic lives, and propose an anti-dote to it.

Of course, this book is also about healing, and about lengthening our life span, but believe me it's not that difficult. Try it yourself.

What's far more challenging and worth our sincere effort is – discovering why you were sent to this planet in the first place.

You would be truly enlightened, the day you discover this answer to this riddle.

Acknowledgment

I would like to thank, 'destiny' and only 'destiny' for giving me the inspiration to write this book. Without 'her' help, I believe, nothing is possible in this world. There are a few self-development techniques mentioned in this book that I can safely claim as 'my own.'

I have personally experienced the free flow of the CNS energy, coursing through my body and kicking in dramatic changes. But owing to a few unfortunate events that unfolded in my life, that you can call 'destiny,' somewhere along the way, I lost all my energy.

To get myself back into good health and to re-activate my dormant energy, I went on a self-exploratory trip, looking for answers to my vexing issues.

That's when I stumbled on a discovery of a few, very ancient techniques, which I started practicing with a lot of interest and vigor, such as 'womb breathing' in Taoist breathing, and surprisingly, these techniques came quite naturally to me, as if I'd been practicing those techniques in all my previous births.

As I mentioned, I had experienced the full force of the CNS energy before through a few meditation techniques, almost instinctively, without knowing that they were mentioned in some ancient texts. I made this startling discovery later.

This was like a revelation! A re-awakening! Something like 'learning' 'un-learning' and 're-learning,' which is the sole reason, I started regarding it as my 'destiny.'

I can't say, I have achieved fully, all that I have set out to achieve, after this –reawakening, but I am on that path.

Presently, I sincerely thank 'destiny' for what I am today, because, as I mentioned earlier, nothing in my life, not even the writing of this book would have been possible, without the mysterious hand of Lady Destiny.

Without her, I would not have experienced the 'pain,' not felt driven to write this treatise.

Table of Contents

Chapter 1

In TCM, there is no concept of a Central Nervous System

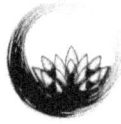

66 An allopathic doctor might say you are perfectly healthy, but you are not!" says Kevin Lau, a practitioner of traditional Chinese medicine, based out of New York's Chinatown.

As a healer, Dr. Lau would follow a completely different approach altogether. He might begin by examining the patient's tongue, followed by an examination of the pulse, or rather the pulses of each one of the patient's 12 organs. And in the end, he would announce the diagnosis— an "energy leak" from the heart, causing nervous palpitations and insomnia!

You might faint at hearing this diagnosis, but Dr Lau would most likely carry on nonchalantly, "You have too many thoughts, clouding your brain vessel. You are unable to drive those out of your brain, even when you go to sleep."

The penny drops and the patient is stunned because Dr. Lau is bang on target!

"What's the remedy?" he inquires. Dr. Lau patiently explains it would require acupuncture, qigong (a form of Chinese yoga), meditation, some dietary amendments and herbal remedies. Also, major lifestyle adjustments. The patient leaves, armed with three main herbal fixes from Dr. Lau, namely - green orange peel, sour date seed and liquorice root, along with a dozen other exotic concoctions.

If Dr Lau comes across as a charlatan to a modern-day business consultant, it's not surprising. The Traditional Chinese Medicine (TCM) is over 2,000 years old, and its roots can be traced back to The Yellow Emperor's Classic of Internal Medicine, which is one of the oldest treatises on conventional Chinese medicine.

Only lately people have begun to discover that some of these old herbal formulae really work, especially against deep-set chronic diseases. The best news is that often TCM works more strongly in areas, where Allopathic medicine is considered weak, i.e., in case of chronic diseases. Or maybe these old tricks of the trade also work in other, less complex cases, but the problem is that no one has ever tried.

The Story of Traditional Chinese Medicine (TCM)

There is no clearly defined, commonly practiced, one system of TCM, so even where the treatment has been found to be highly effective, there is no evidence-based body of research to testify to its effectiveness, against a more established, research-backed system of Western medicine. As a consequence, at best TCM is considered "complementary" and at worst, an "alternate" system of medicine, for patients, who find no hope of a permanent cure in Western medicine, in cases, where only palliative care exists, as with chronic diseases.

Some clues of early TCM practices have been gathered from oracle bones, carved jade and bronze inscriptions, uncovered during excavations of old Chinese civilizations. A lot more detail can be found in the *Inner Canon of the Yellow Emperor* (Huangdi Neijing) dating 1st century BC. And the rest has been added by subsequent practitioners, but have not been properly documented.

Rooted in Balance and Harmony

The root concept in TCM is the balance between yin (female energy) and yang (male energy) and the "five elements" of wood, fire, earth, metal and water, same as in the Indian system of Ayurveda.

The "six pathogens" that have been identified in TCM that cause all kinds of diseases known and unknown to man are cold, wind, dryness, heat, dampness and fire. The "seven emotions" that play a vital role in keeping human beings healthy are joy, anger, anxiety, obsession, sadness, horror and fear – but only if an individual is able to maintain a proper balance between these emotions.

Any kind of an excess, or deficiency in any of these components can cause illness, according to the ancient Chinese medical theory.

Do you drink too much? Talk too much? Exercise too much? Any kind of excess is bad for your health in TCM, so live a life of moderation in order to stay healthy. In addition, in TCM good health requires the pull of a vital life force or energy that the Chinese identify as qi ("chee"). This energy must course smoothly through our body and along the 14 major channels, or "meridians"; or we may report sick. Obstructions in the flow of this energy get manifested as diseases of all kind. Put simply, a malignant tumour in the liver might be interpreted as a "deficiency of the yin in the stomach" or "damp heat affecting the spleen" or "disharmony between the liver and the spleen," in which case your TCM therapist may suggest acupuncture or a herbal formula for the release of "the trapped qi."

Under TCM, organs, and all our bodily processes are inter-linked and they talk to one another. They function as a system, in complete harmony. Things go wrong, only when there is discord or imbalance between them.

The body's qi (the life force or the vital breath) that flows through all the invisible meridians of the body is an essential aspect of the TCM tenets. It forms an energy network, connecting the various organs, nerves, veins, tissues, cells, and atoms, and finally the consciousness itself.

The Meridians

Meridians are complete yet subtle channels of information that connect all the organs and tissues of the body. Although invisible, each of them has their own specific programmes to follow just like radio channels.

The major meridians are 12 in number, and each of these, as per the TCM theory, connect to one of the 12 major organs of the body.

Apart from these there are also other Meridians that relate to a variety of phenomena such as planetary movements, seasons, and circadian rhythms. The information or energy that passes through these meridians, as explained before is qi.

Yin vs. Yang

TCM relies totally on the restoration and maintenance of the delicate yin-yang Balance. These are two opposing, independent forces of the body. While the yin represents all passive, feminine, dark, and receptive attributes, yang represents bright, active, light, and masculine attributes. Every organ of the human body has both yin, as well as, yang qualities, although in all individuals one of these two forces may be more pronounced in some organs and functions, and less in others. For instance, in TCM, the heart is considered a yin organ, and the stomach a yang organ.

Five Organs Network of the Body (Zang Fu)

The heart, kidney, liver, spleen, and lung are the five main organs of a human body. They regulate, store, organize and distribute five vital constituents namely shen, jing, blood, moisture, and qi, all of which are responsible for all our bodily functions.

In Western medicine, these five organs have distinct physical structure, and characteristics but in TCM, they are the functional networks of one, unified body. The function of each of these organ networks is to govern the visceral organs, tissues, functions, associated structures, and also the pathways of qi (Jing Luo, also known as the acupuncture channels) together and in perfect harmony in every healthy human being.

The Heart Network

The Heart, which houses the Shen or mind, is in charge of propelling blood and sustaining the higher functions and faculties of the human body, which includes internal as well as external communication and perception. It is even responsible for regular pulse maintenance and influences the spirit or vitality of an individual. The tongue, the arteries and a person's complexion are all influenced by the Heart network.

The key emotion associated with heart is joy and when this emotion goes out of balance, one might experience mental restlessness, insomnia, depression, confusion, anxiety, despair, fidgeting, and a lack of vitality and enthusiasm. He or she might get startled very easily. Symptoms of an imbalance in the heart region may include irregular heartbeats, poor memory and concentration, excessive dreaming, spontaneous sweating, dizziness, and heart palpitations.

The Kidney Network

The kidney is like the ocean of the body. It stores the Jing or the essence and manages the fluid metabolism. It also governs the will, monitors growth and development, controls reproduction and regeneration, and oversees the functioning of the bones and marrow, brain, lumbar region, teeth, and ears.

The emotion associated with the kidney is fear. When it goes out of balance, the subject may experience fearfulness, insecurity, isolation, aloofness and a lack of willpower. Any imbalance in this organ might lead to symptoms such as frequent urination, urinary incontinence, night sweats, dry mouth, vertigo, poor short-term memory, sore or weak knees, lower back pain, ringing in ears or hearing loss, premature greying of hair or hair loss, osteoporosis and lowered libido.

The Liver Network

The Liver is the storage area of the blood and is in charge of blood circulation in nerves and tendons. It governs the pressure, volume and evenness of the blood and qi circulation and controls judgement and temperament. It also regulates the secretion of bile. The liver network connects the eyes, the nails and the tendons.

The emotion associated with the liver network is anger and when it goes out of balance, one might experience resentment, frustration, moodiness, bitterness, irritability and explosive bouts of anger. The symptoms of liver imbalance include a bitter taste in the mouth, red face, chest distension, dizziness, menstrual problems (heavy or irregular periods with cramps), jaundice, tendonitis, headaches, nausea, vomiting, breast tenderness, sighing, swelling or itching in genitals, dry skin and hair, blurred vision, and floaters.

The Spleen Network

Absorbing of nutrients and transportation are the two key actions that define the functions of the spleen network in TCM. It helps in digesting food and absorbing nutrients, thereby forming blood and qi. It holds blood within the vessels and maintains density, stability and viscosity of tissues and fluids. The spleen network connects muscles, mouth and lips and governs functions, such as studying, thinking, and remembering.

Worry or anxiety is the emotion associated with spleen and when that goes out of balance, one tends to focus or dwell a lot on a particular vexing issue, leading to stress and anxiety. The symptoms of spleen imbalance include exhaustion, loss of appetite, poor digestion, loose stools or diarrhoea, abdominal distension, mucous discharge, pale lips, weak muscles, excessive menstrual blood flow and various other bleeding disorders. The subject may even sustain bruises easily.

The Lung Network

In TCM lung is considered as the master of Qi. Its job is to create qi from the air and then redistribute it throughout the body. The lung is in charge of respiration and controls sweat, as well as body hair. It is the vital part of the immune system and protects the body from bacteria and viruses. In addition, it provides moisture to the skin and keeps it hydrated.

The emotion associated with the lung network is sadness and when it gets out of balance, one can experience extreme sorrow, grief, or detachment, including uncontrolled crying. The symptoms of lung imbalance include fatigue, shortness of breath, cough, runny nose, sore throat, asthma, headache, fever with chills, chest oppression, dry skin, and pale complexion. There is a tendency to catch colds easily if the person experiences an imbalance in the lung network.

The Human Body in Terms of Yin and Yang

In TCM, there are five yin organs and six yang organs in the human body. The Yin organs include the heart, the kidneys, the liver, the spleen, and the lungs. The yang organs comprise of the stomach, gall bladder, large intestine, small intestine, bladder and the triple burner, which is a functional organ with no physical structure.

Qi and blood, the two primary substance of the human body, can also be described in terms of yin and yang. While blood is yin with its moistening and nourishing properties, Qi is yang with its active, energetic, etheric and vitality attributes. Again it's the imbalance of yin and yang that leads to the emergence of any and all diseases. Apart from the nature of the disease, the body's response or the lack of it also can be analysed in terms of yin and yang.

Each and every yin organ in the body can be paired with its yang counterpart, with which it shares its specific meridian pathways, muscles, tissues, as well as the energy-related functions. For example lung (a yin organ) is paired with the large intestine (a yang organ) and any imbalance in the lung, which eventually also reflects in the large intestine. For instance, if a person is facing extreme mood swings and often flits between fear and joy, there is definitely an imbalance between the kidney and the heart. He could be experiencing symptoms such as disturbed sleep, insomnia, dizziness and heart palpitations.

Similarly if a person is experiencing breathing problems, problems with bowel movements, and mood swings between anger and extreme sadness, the imbalance would be between the liver and the lung. A depression characterized by pensive or obsessive thinking, associated with symptoms such as diarrhoea, decreased appetite and heavy bleeding during periods can denote an imbalance between the liver and the spleen.

Ultimately, in TCM the body must also be in harmony with all the natural elements surrounding it. Therefore, the five phases that represent the five elements of our atmosphere, such as wood, fire, earth, metal, and water correspond to the five stage of human transformation, namely birth, growth, maturity, death and rebirth. These life stages are also associated with emotions. For instance, wood is associated with anger, fire with joy, earth with pensiveness, metal with grief, and water with fear. This five-element paradigm is very important in TCM, so much so that the Chinese will immediately assume a liver imbalance in a person who might be throwing a temper tantrum.

A trained TCM practitioner will be able to diagnose the location of the imbalance accurately and treat it through herbal and acupuncture treatments. The imbalance could have to do with an individual's lifestyle, life state or be a consequence of certain events that may have unfolded in his life. With proper diet and exercise one should be able to clear these imbalances. Proper diet refers to the incorporation of five flavours in a well-rounded such as sweet, bitter, spicy, salty and sour, as well as, the five colours such as black, red, white, yellow and green into your meal. By proper exercise TCM practitioners mean the breathing techniques that would help in the free and unobstructed movement of the Qi. These specific breathing techniques include Qi Gong, Yoga, or Tai Chi.

Current and Past Unresolved Emotional Issues

Emotions, in TCM, correlate directly to specific organs of the body and their states of being. The belief is that if the imbalances in the organ are corrected, it will automatically balance the emotion related to that organ. However, there are cases where the emotional imbalance can cause organ imbalance. It is important for a TCM practitioner to understand this difference in order to prevent the recurrence of this problem.

For instance, let us say a person has been experiencing extreme fits of anger and frustration, has problems sleeping, and is suffering from soreness of the eyes, migraines and constipation. This is a clear indication of an imbalance in the Liver which can be completely corrected through herbs and acupuncture. With the treatment the balance will be restored in the liver, leading to a disappearance of the migraines, improvement in sleep and normal bowel movements. Nevertheless, the liver imbalance might return if the person chooses to remain trapped in a stressful job where his colleagues tend to increase his anger and frustration, or if he is dissipating his energy in staving off a nagging wife at home constantly.

TCM is all about flow and balance. Any stagnation or blockage of the flow can lead to a disease that can manifest in any way possible. Current or past emotional issues that have no avenues for release or expression can manifest as physical symptoms and lead to disharmony or disease in the body. Hence, having a healthy emotional life is extremely important for the overall well-being of the body.

Triple Warmer Meridian

Have you heard of San Jiao? It is an ancient Chinese concept used to describe a function rather than a particular organ. Three burners is what San Jiao refers to – the topmost burner comprises of the organs found above the diaphragm, in your thorax, which are mainly concerned with breathing; the organs in the region above the stomach, concerned with digestion, form the middle burner; the organs of the lower abdomen that relate to the gynaecological and urogenital systems constitute the lower burner. All these organs have to work well together for San Jiao to function well. This will allow optimal fluid transportation in the body.

The San Jiao or the triple warmer meridian is located below the Vagus Nerve in the cavum concha. Any disturbance in the internal organs, problems with breathing or digestion, or issues with gynaecological organs or the urinary tract can be a cause of imbalance in the San Jiao. In TCM, you can eliminate heat and itching, reduce swellings, treat chronic constipation and correct problems with organs in ribcage and abdomen, by restoring and maintaining the balance of the San Jiao.

Functions of the Three Burners

The Upper Burner: The primary function of the upper burner is to distribute the body fluids through the action of the lungs. Known generally as the mist, the upper burner keeps the respiratory system lubricated by transforming the body's energy into vapour. This vapour also moisturises the skin and prohibits the pathogens from invading the body, thereby acting as an important immunity guard. Our skin is our physical shield against all bacteria and viruses and defends us against airborne illnesses.

The Middle Burner: Digestion is the prime function of the middle burner. The spleen and the stomach in the middle burner break down the food, separating the absorbable part from the excretal one. Known generally as the maceration chamber, middle burner ensures the nourishment is garnered well and transported optimally throughout the system.

The Lower Burner: Known as the drainage ditch, the lower burner is in charge of separating fluids for excretion by way of urine. The functioning of the kidney, the urinary bladder, and the small intestine – all come under the lower burner.

Triple Burner Pathology

Upper Burner: The impairment of the misting function of the upper burner is an indication that our defences are breaking down. It generally leads to a cold with symptoms like runny nose, sneezing, sore throat, body aches, and fever. Depending on the location, we may also experience pain behind the ears, earache, sore throat, cheek swelling, or pain in the optic canthus.

Middle Burner: The impairment of the macerating function of the middle burner indicates an imbalance in digestion. You may experience food retention issues such as nausea, heartburn, bloating or excessive belching.

Lower Burner: The impairment of the drainage ditch can lead to issues with urination and water retention. Lower leg edema, urinary retention, burning urination, frequent urination, and loss of bladder control are a few imbalances involving the triple burner.

A proper understanding of the triple burner can help massage therapists to impact a few complex body imbalances healthfully. As a system for the creation, processing and elimination of fluids, the pathology of the triple burner is fascinating rather than mysterious.

Dan Tian or Dan Tien Force

Dan is the force that nourishes the universe at all times. Daoists' believe that this energy exists in people the same way as it exists in the universe, especially in a special areas known as Dan Tians.

Dan Tian refers to an area in the lower abdomen, which is located about three finger width below the naval and two finger width behind the naval. This is where the jing is stored. It is represented as uterus in women and chamber of essence in men.

In Taoist Texts, there are three Dan Tians. The first one is the lower Dan Tian as mentioned above. The second one or the middle Dan Tian is the one that is at the level of the heart, which stores the qi. The upper Dan Tian is the brain or the sea of marrow and it lies at the central point just higher than the eye brows and co-related with the spirit and/or the higher consciousness.

By concentrating on the Dan Tian, you can become aware of your entire body, which is why it is called as the physical center. Dan Tian being a power house of energy, many Tai Chi practitioners and martial artists focus on the area, during intense practice, in order to ignite their entire body.

All About Mingmen

The Mingmen or the Gate of Life as it's called is the area that is located on the middle of the lower back. This is where the genuine yin and yang of the body is found. This is from where all the substances and functions of the body develop. A healthy Mingmen supplies adequate amount of warmth to the body, which is why it is called the Gate of Vitality.

Through the three heaters - the upper, middle, and lower ones – the Gate of Vitality provides us with adequate amount of warmth to help us stay alive. The original energy for this fire comes from our genes. We begin to draw on it after birth. The energy that is created from consuming food to replenish it.

The Gate of Life is also known as the Mansion of Water and Fire, The Sea of Essence and qi, the Nest of Life and Death, and the house of Yin and Yang. If depleted and damaged, it can disconnect the five solid organs and six hollow organs, leading to a massive imbalance of Yin and Yang, which then manifests into various disease forms.

In this context, a very old definition of Mingmen, "The Gate of Life is the sum of the two kidneys." The two kidneys here are the yin kidney and the yang kidney. It encompasses the yin and yang functions of the entire body.

The yang function of the Mingmen is very evident in the digestive process. In the traditional Chinese physiology, the digestive fire determines the strength of the digestion. If this fire is strong enough the food that we consume can be efficiently transformed into blood and qi.

If weak, it will fail to provide the necessary warmth, thereby manifesting as diarrhoea, loose stools, bloating and various other signs of digestive disorders. Among the many methods, Energetics (Qi Gong) and Herbalism are the two best ways to strengthen the Mingmen.

Chapter 2

Tibetan 'Fountain of Youth' Exercises

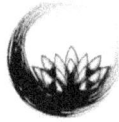

If you want to turn back the clock and enjoy being at the peak of your health, try the Five Tibetan Rites.

It's a set of five exercises, performed up to 21 times, which are believed to have miraculous healing powers and age-defying benefits. Tibetan monks discovered the Rites, nearly two thousand years, ago and that's the secret to their youthful appearance.

The monks claim that the set of five exercises have the power to stimulate all glands of our endocrine system that control and trigger the ageing process in human beings. An imbalance in these glands and the hormones produced by them, in Buddhist philosophy can also impact the body's seven *chakras*, and any imbalance at any of those seven *chakras* can cause other acute or chronic ailments, as well.

How to Perform These Exercises

Although you are required to perform the exercises 21 times, it's recommended that you initially go slow and steady. For starters, begin the routine by doing just five repetitions of each exercise, each day.

Contraindication: Don't attempt the exercises if you have any back, wrist or neck-related issues. Listen to your body and give yourself a break if you have any kind of pain in your knee joints or lower back. Set a pace that your body demands, until you are more accustomed to the rigors of this demanding exercise.

However practiced daily, the five exercises will set you on the path to rejuvenation and the discovery of a youthful energy in you.

First Tibetan - Rite #1

Stand upright with your arms outstretched horizontal to the floor, palms facing down and arms in line with your shoulders, straight as a ramrod. Now turn around clockwise. Gradually increase the number of turns from 1 to 21.

Relax.

Second Tibetan - Rite #2

Lie flat on the floor, face up. Fully extend your arms along your sides and press your hands against the floor. Then raise your head off the floor, while pressing your chin into your chest. As you do this, lift your legs, knees straight, into a vertical position. Just be careful not to let your knees bend in this position. Now slowly lower your legs and head to the floor, while mindful of not bending your knees. After holding this position for a few seconds, allow your muscles to relax before repeating the cycle.

Exhale...

Third Tibetan - Rite #3

Kneel on the floor, while keeping your body straight.

Place your hands on the backs of your thigh muscles. Incline your head and bring your neck forward, pressing your chin against your chest.

Then throw your head back, while arching your spine. As you arch, you can hold your thighs for support. Remember to keep your toes curled, while doing this exercise.

Exhale...

Fourth Tibetan - Rite #4

Sit down on the floor with your legs stretched right in front of you. Keeping your body straight, place the palms of your hands on the floor, parallel to your buttocks.

Then press your chin forward against the chest. Next drop the head backward as far as it will go, while at the same time raising your body in a manner that the knees bend but the arms remain straight. Constrict and feel tension in every big or small muscle of your body.

Now relax your muscles and breathe out, before repeating the cycle.

Fifth Tibetan - Rite #5

Stretch your arms perpendicular to the floor, while keeping the spine curved. Now throw your head back as far as it would go. Next, bend slightly at the hips in a manner that your body is in an inverted "V" position. Last, throw the chin forward, pressing it against the chest. Exhale...

Benefits of Rites

Practicing these rites daily will improve your blood circulation, and give relief from a lot of acute and chronic ailments. They will also clear out disturbing thoughts, disturbed sleep patterns and cure migraines etc. The rites encourage energy production, elevate moods, boosts our immune system and can correct diseases of the prostrate and menopausal symptoms. They also have a positive impact on acidity, indigestion and intestine-related issues and improve lymphatic circulation in the body.

In the end it doesn't or shouldn't matter if the fountain of youth is a real or a metaphorical expression. What matter is that if it improves your experience of life; why not explore its benefits?

Tibetan Rejuvenation Rite #6

The series of five Tibetan exercises described above can be practiced two or three times a day, but the following exercise, according to the learned Tibetan Lamas is a restrictive exercise with a very special purpose and it ought to be practiced only in special circumstances that we will explain in a while.

If you are not practicing the first five exercises regularly, we repeat, do not practice this exercise. We forewarn you.

This is because, the main purpose of the Tibetan #6 exercise is to channelize the excess sexual/reproductive energy generated by the activity of the base chakra (referred to as vortexes) to all the other higher chakras along the spine, especially to the brow chakra, which regulates spiritual awakening and psychic abilities.

Experts recommend the use of this exercise only when a native experiences excessive sexual urge, otherwise this exercise is known to do more harm than good, by draining the energy from the base chakra.

On the flip side, by routinely practicing the first five Tibetan exercises, explained in detail in this Chapter, it's possible to raise the energy of the base chakra to a level, where the sexual urge can be calmed and balanced with all other desires. This ability can be acquired anytime, regardless of the native's age.

How is Tibetan #6 Different?

As mentioned earlier, this Rite is remarkably different from all the previously described Tibetan exercises. Firstly, it's one of the easiest to perform from the physical perspective, and second, it involves breath control, a prolonged holding of the breath, which takes practice to perfect. The third difference is that after each cycle of Tibetan #6, you are required to repeat several cycles of deep breathing. One final difference is that no more than three repeats are recommended of Tibetan Rite #6 for an average person.

The sequence of Tibetan #6 is as follows:

✓ Stand straight and breathe out completely.
✓ Bend over forward and place your hands on your knees, while exhaling every trace of air from your lungs
✓ With your lungs empty return to the standing position

✓ Place your hands on your waist and push your shoulders up by pressing down with your hands. Pull your abdomen in as much as possible and raise your chest to completely empty your lungs
✓ Hold this position as long as you can
✓ Breathe in slowly through your nose to once again fill your lungs
✓ Exhale through the mouth, while letting your arms hang free
✓ Take several deep breaths before repeating this cycle

Once again, please understand that in order to perform rite number six, it is absolutely necessary that the native have an active sexual interest. It is absolutely impossible, rather meaningless for a person to perform this rite if he has no sexual urge, to begin with. Such as person shouldn't even attempt to do it, as it would only lead to harm than benefit.

Instead, such an individual, regardless of age ought to concentrate on practicing only the first five rites until he regains a normal sexual urge.

Chapter 3

The Chakra System

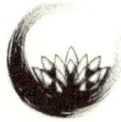

In Hindu mythology, every human body has an invisible copy made up of tiny droplets of energy. It is located about two to five centimetres in front and around your body and surrounds it like a halo.

This halo of energy is connected to our physical body with seven major pipes, called the chakras, which are invisible to the naked eye. Each chakra is assigned a different, specialized task and each has its own special rainbow colors – Red, Orange, Yellow, Green, Blue, Indigo and Violet. As color is light and has a frequency of its own, each chakra color represents the rate at which each chakra vibrates and functions.

Chakras and their Colours
Root Chakra
Sacral Chakra
Solar Plexus
Heart Chakra
Throat Chakra
Third eye Chakra
Crown Chakra

The Constant Whirring Wheel

"*Chakra*" is a Sanskrit word, meaning the "wheel." These energy filters were named because of their resemblance to the spinning wheel, which is not physically present, but which Hindu scholars believe exist in the ethereal body that cannot be seen or touched, or even filmed and spotted with an X-ray, but which can be sensed only through higher faculties.

The number seven is mythical and has immense significance. Conical shaped, the seven main *chakras* align along the vertical axis of the body, from the last vertebra of the spine to the top of the head.

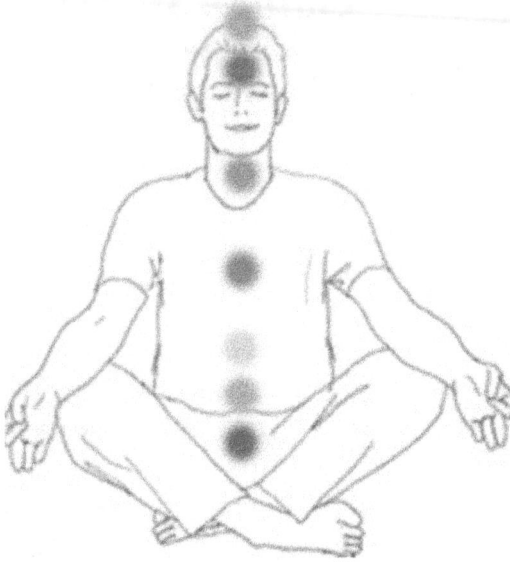

Put simply, a chakra may metaphorically be a wheel or a vortex, but it operates like a spinning ball of energy, concentrated at that particular point. These chakras are vital links between the endocrine and the nervous system.

As such, each chakra corresponds to an endocrine gland and also, a bunch of nerves, identified as the plexus, which makes them important seats of spiritual healing.

Chakras Link the Physical with the Metaphysical

Chakras are believed to regulate the flow of energy through electric nodes (meridians) that course through our body. The chakras circuit sometimes gets blocked because of stress or disease that begin to obstruct this free flow of energy, leading to various symptoms, depending upon the chakra involved.

Clearing and opening the clogged chakras is called 'chakra balancing' or 'chakra healing' which leads to emotional, physical and spiritual well-being of an individual. Regular meditation activates these chakras.

The following chart maps out the primary qualities of each *chakra*, its corresponding location in the body, color, physical and emotional realms of influence, and significance.

Chakra 1 - The Base or the Root Chakra

Flaming red in colour, it's located at the perineum, i.e. the base of the spine. Associated with the legs, feet, bones, large intestine and adrenal glands, any imbalance here is likely to cause issues related with arthritis, knee pain, sciatica, eating disorders, and constipation. On an emotional plane, it may reflect as paranoia, fear, procrastination and defensiveness.

In *Tantra Shastra*, we have a bundle of dormant energy resting like a coiled serpent at the base of the spine. When this dormant energy is awakened through meditation, energy begins to flow upward through the seven chakras, leading to a heightened sense of consciousness. This is known as *kundalini* awakening. Most mortal beings live and die, without making the effort of self-realization through *kudalini* awakening, which can transport them to another realm, altogether.

When the root chakra is balanced, one feels protected, supported and grounded to the physical world.

The lesson of this chakra is self-preservation; we have to live in the here and now. There is one syllable mantra associated with each chakra. Chanting these mantras will facilitate the release of energy from that chakra. The root chakra's seed mantra is LAM, standing for element earth.

Healing Root Chakra

Since it's the densest chakra of all, intense physical activities can open up this clogged chakra. Aromatherapy, also works with this chakra, besides the use of gemstones, as this chakra symbolizes the earth element. Gardening is also beneficial for the healing of the root chakra.

Chakra 2 - The Sacral Chakra

This orange coloured chakra, also known as the Hara chakra is located in the pelvic region. It controls functions of the lower abdomen, kidneys, bladder, circulatory system and reproductive organs and glands. This chakra rules emotions and manifests its energy in the form of desire, pleasure, sexuality, procreation and creativity. Blocked energy can erupt in emotional problems, compulsive or obsessive behaviour and sexual guilt.

One school of thought is that through martial arts and the practice of Tai Chi, it's possible to expand the hara chakra, leading to a sudden release of energy (chi in Chinese), accompanied by a feeling of well-being.

When this chakra is balanced, the native is courageous, is a risk-taker, highly creative and committed. An extrovert, he or she also has a strong sexual desire.

The lesson of this chakra is to honour others.

Healing Sacral Chakra

Tantric yoga and hip poses are good exercises to activate this chakra. The foods that work with this chakra are citrus fruits like oranges, also mangoes and pumpkins, as this chakra is wired to the water element and the mantra for activation of this chakra is VAM.

Chakra 3 – The Solar Plexus or the Naval Chakra

Yellow in colour, the Solar chakra lies a few inches above the navel in the solar plexus area. This is connected with the digestive system, muscles, pancreas and adrenals. It's considered the emotional power house. Feelings of ambition, drive, power, laughter, joy and anger are derived from the Solar Plexus. Blockage may result in anger, frustration, lack of drive, and an acute sense of victimhood. When the chakra is well-balanced, the native has high self-esteem, confidence and also compassion for others.

The lesson of this chakra is self-acceptance.

Healing Solar Plexus Chakra

Yantras work very well with this chakra. This chakra regulates logical thinking, numerical and reasoning ability. It's associated with all kind of cognitive tasks. Sun bathing is recommended for this chakra, as it corresponds to the fire element and the mantra for its activation is RAM. Any confidence-building measure strengthens the third chakra, such as public speaking exercises. Breathing exercises are also good for the solar plexus.

Chakra 4 – The Heart Chakra

Jade-green in colour, this chakra's seat is the human heart. Blockages in this chakra can cause asthma, heart and lung disease, issues with the breasts, lymphatic system, upper back and shoulder problems, arm and wrist pain.

Emotional imbalances include jealousy, anger, frustration, loneliness and bitterness. When this chakra is balanced we feel joy, gratitude, love, compassion, forgiveness, brotherhood and trust.

The lesson of this chakra is love.

Blockage can reveal themselves in dysfunctional immune system, lung and heart-related ailments, criminal tendencies.

Healing the Fourth Chakra

Touch therapy is very good for activating this chakra. Hugging–even self-hugging works. Since this chakra corresponds to the air element, breathing exercises and the simple act of deep inhalation and exhalation of oxygen-rich air will cause the release of toxins and unblock this chakra. The mantra for activation of this 'air' chakra is YAM.

Chakra 5 -The Throat Chakra

Turquoise in colour, this chakra is located in the thoracic region. It rules communication, creativity, self-expression and judgment. Connected to the neck, shoulders, arms, hands, thyroid and the parathyroid glands, it regulates hearing, ideation, self-healing, transformation and purification.

Blockage can reflect in creative blocks, dishonesty or communication-related problems,

When balanced, the person has the gift of the gab, is a very good orator, and articulates his ideas and thoughts very well. These natives also have high integrity and make good listeners too.

The element for this chakra is Ether and the mantra is HAM.

The lesson of this chakra is to speak up and let yourself be heard.

Healing Fifth Chakra

Music therapy is extremely effective with these natives. Healing can also take the form of chanting mantras, humming an old song, singing hymns, etc.

Chakra 6 – The Third Eye or the Brow Chakra

Indigo in colour, this chakra is located at the centre of the forehead between the eyebrows, where Indian married women, put their *bindi*, and the Hindu men put the *tilak* mark. This is the site of spiritual awakening. This chakra rules inner vision, intuition, knowledge, spiritual quest and wisdom. All dreams for this life and recollections of the past lie embedded in this Chakra. Blockage can appear as memory-related disorders and depression.

Well balanced, the native is clear-headed, wise, intuitive and focused, and can effectively differentiate between truth and falsehood.

The lesson of this chakra is to be a visionary. The element for this chakra is Light and mantra is OM.

Healing the Sixth Chakra

Techniques of visualization and dream therapy work best with this chakra. Regular meditation is also extremely helpful. The idea is to relax and pin your gaze inwards. There is a whole universe to be explored there as well.

Chakra 7 – The Crown Chakra

Violet in colour, this chakra lies at approximately four finger width above the head, beneath the Fontanelle (space between the bones of the skull in an infant or fetus), which is often visible in a new-born child. This chakra gives us access to higher consciousness.

The crown chakra is aligned to the cerebral cortex, the central nervous system and the pituitary gland. It is concerned with information, understanding, acceptance and the experience of bliss. This chakra rules divine purpose and human destiny. Blockage can result in psychiatric problems and mental health issues.

When balanced, the native is content and has unshakeable faith in justice and mercy. The element for this chakra is 'beyond elements' and mantra is Silent OM.

The lesson of this chakra is 'Be aware.'

Healing Chakra Seven

Meditation – of any kind – works beautifully for this chakra. Just relax and open yourself to the Universe in a void and be a silent observer. It works.

CHAKRA CHART ©

	Root Muladhara Support	Sacral Svadhisthana Dwelling Place	Solar Plexus Manipura Jeweled City	Heart Anahata Unstruck Sound	Throat Vishuddha Noble Purity	Third Eye Ajna To Know	Crown Sahasrara Thousandfold
Location	Base of spine Legs Bones Immune System	Pelvis Low back Abdomen Ovaries Prostate	Solar Plexus Pancreas Adrenals	Heart Lungs & Arms Thymus	Throat Mouth Ears Hands Thyroid	Brow Between Eyebrows Pineal Pituitary	Top of head
Element	Earth	Water	Fire	Air	Ether / Sound	Mind / Light	Beyond elements
Crystals	Garnet Red Jasper	Moonstone Carnelian	Citrine Tigers Eye	Rose Quartz Aventurine	Blue Lace Agate Angelite	Sodalite Lapis	Clear Quartz Amethyst
Goddess Archetype	Kali Durga, Shakti Artemis	Bharani Aphrodite	Lakshmi Ariadne	Sita, Tara Hera	Saraswati Athena	Gayatri Hecate	Radha Isis
Emanating Color	Red	Orange	Yellow	Green	Blue	Indigo	Violet White
Balancing Color	Green	Blue	Violet	Red			
Identity	Physical Self-Preservation	Emotional Self-Gratification	Ego Self-Definition	Social Self-Acceptance	Creative Self-Expression	Archetypal Self-Reflection	Universal Self-Knowledge
Lesson	To have, To be here	To feel, To want, To create	To act	To love & Be loved	To create, To speak & be heard	To see, To witness	To know.
Rights and Responsibilities							
Balanced Chakra Energy	Feels safe and secure. Physically healthy. Good body image. Right livelihood Prosperous. Lives in here & now. Able to be still.	Emotional intelligence. Can change. Can nurture self & others. Healthy boundaries. Can feel pain & pleasure. Sexual satisfaction.	Self-confident. Good self esteem. Right action. Healthy boundaries. Takes responsibility. Disciplined. Creative. Sense of belonging.	Loving Caring Shows compassion. Accepting. Loving to self & others. Peaceful Content. Centered. Trusting. Non-judgment.	Voice that is full, resonant Communicates clearly with others. Good self-expression. Good listener. Truthful Creative expression.	Keen intuition. Imaginative. Good memory. Good dream recall. Has guiding vision for life Able to watch and "witness." Can see the big picture.	Spiritually connected. Wisdom & mastery. Intelligence. Presence. Able to question. Able to assimilate & analyze info. Open Mind.

26

Challenges	Fear	Guilt	Shame	Grief	Deceit	Illusion	Attachment
Excessive Chakra Energy	Sluggish. Heaviness. Monotony. Hoarding. Materialistic. Greedy. Workaholic.	Too sensitive. Obsessive. Poor boundaries. Emotional dependency. Emotional instability. Sensual/sexual addictions.	Domineering. Blaming. Aggressive. Fighty. Hyperactive. Competitive.	Codependent (too much focus on others). Poor boundaries. Jealousy. Being a martyr. Being a pleaser.	Excessive talking. Poor listener. Over extended. Gossiping. Too loud. Unable to keep secret. Forced creative expression.	Trouble concentrating. Headaches. Intrusive memories. Excessive fantasizing. Nightmares. Obsession. Delusion.	Too intellectual. Spiritual/Religious addiction. Confusion. Detachment from spirit. Dissociation from body. Living "in your head."
Deficient Chakra Energy	Fear/Anxiety. Lacks discipline. Restless. Spacey. Difficulty manifesting. Resists structure.	Emotional numbness. Fear of pleasure. Fear of change. Apathetic. Bored. Rigidity. Impotence.	Weak will. Poor self-esteem. Submissive. Sluggish. Fearful. Lacking energy.	Antisocial. Withdrawn. Critical. Intolerant. Lonely. Isolated. Lacking empathy.	Fear of speaking. Poor rhythm. Weak voice. Excessive shyness. Denial of creative expression.	Unimaginative. Inattentive. Poor memory. Poor vision. Cannot see patterns. Denial. Inflexible thinking.	Trouble learning. Spiritual uncertainty. Limited beliefs. Materialism. Apathetic. Closed mind.
Musical Note	C Drum	D Brass	E Sax	F Violin	G Flute	A Crystal bowl	B Voice
Bija Mantra (Increase & Attract)	Lam As in "Lum"	Vam As in "Vum"	Ram "Rum" with rolling R.	Yam As in "Yum"	Ham As in "Hum"	Om	Beyond sound
Vowel sounds (Distribute)	O As in "toe"	OO As in "moo"	Ah As in "awe"	A As in "play"	EE As in "speak"	Mmmm	Silence or NG As in "sing"
Breathing Practices	Dirgha breath (Complete breath)	Dirgha breath (Complete breath)	Kapalabhati (Breath of fire)	Nadi Shodhana (Alternate nostril)	Ujjayi breath (Ocean Breath)	Kapalabhati	Nadi Shodhana (Alternate nostril) Nadi Shodhana

Continued

27

CHAKRA CHART ©	Root Muladhara	Sacral Svadhisthana Dwelling Place	Solar Plexus Manipura Jeweled City	Heart Anahata	Throat Vishuddha Noble Purity	Third Eye Ajna To Know	Crown Sahasrara Thousandfold
Yoga Postures	Foot & leg stretches. Seated lying & standing poses. Core lift. Forward fold. Locust. Child. Lie face down.	Cobra. Cat stretches. Seated hip openers. Core lift. Bound angle. Standing hip circles & stretches. Eagle or cow legs.	Core lift. Abdominal exercises. Sun salute. Warrior 1. Twists. Boat / Cobra. Restorative backbends. Spinal twist. Forward fold.	Chest & shoulder openers. Backbends to increase energy. Forward bends to decrease. Fish. Cobra. Bridge	Neck and shoulder stretches. Bridge. Shoulder stand. Half shoulder stand. Fish (supported). Fish. Camel.	Eye exercises. Gazing. Close eyes. Spinal twist. Yoga Mudra.	Inversions. Headstand. Yoga Mudra.
Other Healing Activities	Walking. Hiking. Play. Garden. Right eating & sleeping. Work with hands.	Bathe. Swim. Improve flexibility. Dance. Enjoy your senses. Experience emotions.	Get moving. Take risks. Release anger & attachments. Nurture self. Laugh. Balance w/ light or dark.	Breath work. Animals. practice self-acceptance of self & others. Forgiveness. Gratitude. Love.	Chanting. Singing. Being silent. Listen to or create music. Be creative. Journal. Eat fruits.	Meditate. Enjoy and create beauty. Journal. Create visual art. Visual stimulation.	Meditate. Pray. Learn & create. Experience beauty. Use your brainpower. Define beliefs & values.

Chapter 4

Acupressure & Acupuncture

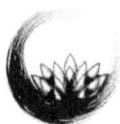

Very often, people tend to associate acupuncture with TCM. Although acupuncture is a very integral part of TCM, TCM also comprises of several other therapeutic interventions, such as acupressure, cupping, magnet therapy, moxibustion, and various massage techniques such as tuina and guasha.

The Meridian Connection

In TCM, 12 meridians enable the Qi to flow through the body. These meridians exist in pairs, each of them having their own acupuncture/acupressure point along the paths. For instance, there are about 21 points in the Spleen Meridian, 9 in the Heart Meridian, 14 in the Liver Meridian, and 27 in the Kidney Meridian.

Each meridian is associated with one organ, which can be either yin (female) or yang (male). Qi flowing across the meridians is very much like water flowing across a stream. If there are any obstructions, the flow can get clogged. Within the human body, such obstructions could be poor nutrition, stress, or even an injury. Any blockage in the meridian can lead to the body experiencing disorders in the area. The only way to restore the natural flow of Qi, is to identify and remove the blockage or obstruction.

Both acupuncture as well as acupressure are based on the concept of the flow of Qi. Both use physical pressure to clear blockages in meridians, thereby helping the person heal. Such pressure can make the brain release certain chemicals (endorphins) that tend to muffle the pain signals and help the person enjoy pleasurable feelings. With the tension receding, the blood starts flowing more freely and the body begins to find its balance.

The road map of acupoints that acupuncture and acupressure use is the same. Acupoints are the energy hot spots along the meridians where in the energy collects, giving better access to Qi. In acupuncture, these points are assessed by needles; while in acupressure these are assessed through the less-invasive method of touch.

By manipulating the acupoints, one can increase or decrease the flow of Qi along a particular meridian.

Points on Hands/Feet and on the Whole Body

There are hundreds of acupoints in the human body. Similar to the electrical outlets, they make it easier to access the electrical charge of the underlying meridian. You can recognize them as indentations. For instance, the hollow that you find at your temples is an acupoint. The notch that exists between the top of the sternum and the collarbone is also an acupoint.

TCM practitioners use this complex acupuncture points' chart to diagnose and treat their patients. The chart originally identified 365 points, a number that corresponded to the total number of days in a calendar year. Lately, additional points have been identified and the channels between them recognized.

It often takes years for TCM practitioners to memorize the location of each acupoint. But there are a few points that are considered the power players. Most of these are found at the crossroads of the meridians. Manipulating these points can provide immense benefits to multiple organ systems.

Each acupoint has been assigned a code that is a combination of a letter and a number corresponding to the point's location in the body. It also has a poetic name derived from its Chinese character, which is also based on its location or the benefit accruing from pressing that point.

Mingmen Point – Location, Functions and its Healing Properties

As discussed in our earlier chapter, there is hardly any point that is more exalted than the Gate of Life, or *Mingmen*. It is a very powerful point that goes up to the core of our existence or life. It provides access to the gate from which we emerge with all our essence, constitution, and destiny. It is this point that can help us fulfill our destiny and realize our fullest potential.

Mingmen is an energy center that is located in our lower torso. It is associated with three acupuncture points namely the Governing Vessel 4 (Gv4), Conception Vessel 4 (Cv4) and Conception Vessel 5 (Cv5). If you can access the shallow point at the center of your lower back, between the third and the fourth lumbar vertebrae, you should be able to locate your Gv4. It is almost at the same level as the navel.

Because of its powerful implications, Mingmen is termed as a remarkable point for revitalization. While reconnecting us with our essence, it also supports us to achieve our highest potential, while raising us to an entirely new level of consciousness. This is the one that help us connect with our original nature.

Positioned between the kidney shu points (BL 23) on the spine, the Mingmen notifies the Kidney Qi powerfully. It supports the water element, thus treating the heat as well as cold conditions of the body.

The problems that can be resolved by manipulating the Mingmen include fever and chills, incontinence, urinary problems, and feeling cold all over the body, especially in areas such as the belly and the lower back. The point can also be used to address reproductive disorders including infertility, irregular menstruation, menstrual pain, impotence, and frigidity. Apart from these, other conditions such as haemorrhoids, prolapse of rectum, poor memory, and tinnitus can also be cured by manipulating the Mingmen. Besides, it also reduces pain in the lower back, stopping it from radiating to the abdomen.

Chapter 5

Everything About Qigong

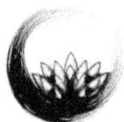

Huang Di Nei Jing, the ancient Chinese medical text book and Yellow Emperor's Inner Canon, the fundamental doctoral thesis of TCM have mentioned Qigong as an integral part of the ancient Chinese Medical system.

Qigong is a type of a gentle exercise that involves repetitive movements and stretches that increase fluid movement and build awareness of the way in which the body moves through space.

Benefits of Qigong

Qigong, as used in Chinese medicine and acupuncture, is aimed at opening the flow of energy along the meridians. Apart from enhancing our ability to feel the life force, it also deepens our communication with Qi.

The slow and gentle movements of Qigong warms the ligaments, muscles, and tendons, tones the vital organs as well as the connective tissues, and also promotes the circulation of fluids such as blood, lymph and synovial across the body.

Types of Qigong Practice

There are mainly two types of Qigong practice:

- **Wai Dan** or the External Elixir that focuses on physical movement as well as concentration
- **Nei Dan** or the Internal Elixir that is about meditation and guided visualization (imagery)

The Techniques of Qigong

The first thing that beginners will learn in Qigong is physical movements that are coordinated with specific breathing techniques. They involve sets of exercises to be practiced each day, until each and every posture or movement is perfected. The exercises are very similar to that of Tai Chi. Once their postures and movements are perfect, they start finding the subtle flow of energy in their movements, postures, transitions, and breathing patterns, and start recognizing fluctuations, if any. That's why the second name for this technique is 'Moving Meditation.'

A few postures in these exercises are similar to those in Yoga and are to be held for longer periods of time. Practicing these postures can help increase the flow of energy and strengthen the limbs. The category that these postures fall into is called **Still Meditation.**

More on Tai Chi

Originating more than two thousand years ago, Tai Chi is the healing art of China. It brings in a lot of health benefits and improves the health conditions of people of all ages, through a series of circular, slow, relaxed, smooth-flowing, and continuous movements.

Tai Chi is about certain theories of movement, specific posture alignment, and also includes one or two specific breathing techniques that generate and circulate tremendous amount of Qi throughout the body. When compared to Qigong, Tai Chi attracts many more practitioners through the sheer fluidity of its movements.

As per Taoism, everything in this world is composed of two opposing yet complementary forces of yin and yang that strike a perfect balance, while working in a relationship. The exercises in Tai Chi are meant to strike this balance between these yin and yang elements, thus making these opposite forces well-aligned to each other and remarkably effective.

A moving form of meditation, Tai Chi includes controlled breathing and precision movements, synchronized in a way to help the practitioner flow with the direction of the Chi (energy), both in as well as around the body.

To a beginner, Qigong may look a lot alike Tai Chi, and while there is significant similarity between the two; but there are also quite a few differences. For instance, Tai Chi is actually a martial art that can be used for healing. On the other hand, Qigong is not really a martial art. It has its exclusive focus on healing.

Tai Chi vs. Qigong - The Essential Differences

We enumerate a few qualitative differences:

1. The Power in Tai Chi is dense, while it is light in Qigong. The forms of Tai Chi are very intricate, especially at the higher level. The Qi that manifests within each of these forms comprises of certain subtle characteristics that have the power to be transformed along with every form. On the other hand, Qigong forms are not so intricate. Also the Qi that is expressed is a lot more general, with less-defined characteristics.

2. The effect of Qi in Tai Chi (at a higher level) is tremendously powerful as it flows along a continuous stream, accumulated strongly throughout the ligaments, tendons, and the meridians. The effect of the Qi in Qigong is considerably less powerful when compared to Tai Chi.

3. Unlike the art of Qigong, the art of Tai Chi is an elaborate and advanced form of choreography.

4. There is no need for a practitioner of Qigong to study the forms. All he has to do is focus on cultivating the Qi. Nevertheless, the practice of Tai Chi is centered solely on the forms, with focus on different aspects such as coordination, integration, precision, unity, connection, and alignment. The Qi that manifests is a result of this form.

5. The meditation that is involved in the art of Qigong is very profound and can make the practitioner go deep into the realm of consciousness.

As opposed to this, the moving meditation, which is the art of Tai Chi, is not so intense.

6. A particular type of Qigong meditation enables the practitioner to achieve a potent healing power that he can use to treat his illness or that of others. In comparison to this, moving Qigong and Tai Chi seem to be less powerful and can be used for one's own overall wellbeing. If you are suffering from ailments such as fever, cold or flu, it is advisable not to practice Tai Chi or Qigong until you recover completely.

More About Tai Chi

Tai Chi is a complex form of art. It can't be described in one, simple sentence. It can be different things for different people. Tai Chi exercise is made up of a series of graceful movements that are accompanied with slow and deep diaphragmatic breathing patterns. The exercise is usually performed while standing.

Deep breathing and meditation are integral parts of Tai Chi, which encourage internal calming and peacefulness. They also help in cleansing stale air. Apart from these, the techniques also help in relaxing the muscles and relieving tension.

Unlike other forms of physical activities, Tai Chi demands a lot of focus, which is very important for meditation. Yang, Wu and Chen are some of the notable forms of Tai Chi. All of these involve slow, deliberate, and graceful movements that flow seamlessly into one another, without any kind of hesitation or obstruction.

Benefits of Tai Chi

Regular practice of Tai Chi can lead to several benefits, such as

* Better body balance that can prevent falls
* Reduction in pain, stiffness and fatigue
* Increase in strength and endurance
* Better aerobic capacity
* Elimination of stress
* Improved psychological health

Apart from the above, Tai Chi can also add to the benefits of cognitive behavioral therapy by improving mental clarity and focus, lowering stress, and increasing positive thoughts. Along with physical exercise, Tai Chi can be described as a form of meditation on wheels.

Reverse Breathing

Our body employs several types of breathing techniques that keeps changing throughout the year, and with every emotional state that we embrace, at every phase of our lives. One such type of breathing is the Reverse Breathing or the Taoist Reverse Breathing.

In this type of breathing you reverse the natural in-out movement of your abdomen. With every inhalation you shrink your belly and with every exhalation you expand it. It is also known as womb or pre-birth breathing, since this is the form of breathing babies adopt when they are in the womb.

The main purpose behind Taoist Reverse Breathing is to help you become aware of and control the subtle physical as well as energetic movements of your body, making sure they coordinate with the rhythm of your breathing. This way every part and function of your body, your etheric body, and your aura, will move in coordination, with every expansion and contraction of your belly.

The Taoist reverse breathing is known to open up, strengthen and stabilize the aura. It is integral to a particular aspect of Lao Tse's "Breathing from the Heels," which is considered the only complete breathing process within Taoism.

Although it is immensely beneficial, reverse breathing should not be done unless one is comfortable practicing the technique of natural abdominal breathing. People who attempt reverse breathing before achieving this level of comfort, can end up tensing their faces, necks and chests, and drawing in their diaphragms upward during inhalation. Apart from negating the positive effects of practice, this can also lead to problems such as diarrhea, chest pain, energy stagnation, hypertension, and increase in heartbeat. It might also lead to emotional and mental confusion, eventually, scattering the energy of awareness.

Chapter 6

Everything About Qi or Chi

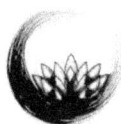

Qi or Chi is the idea of a universal source of energy. It's the energy that is the source of all life.

Without Qi, there can be no life form on planet earth, or elsewhere in the Universe.

It would not be an exaggeration to say that everything around us – is Qi.

In Chinese philosophy, every object, every life form around us comprised of Qi.

It may express itself in various forms in various entities – living or non-living – but this living, conscious, loving intelligence exists in all and, if channelized properly helps us to fulfill our life's purpose.

In short, it gives meaning to our existence on this planet.

The concept of Qi lies at the nucleus of Traditional Chinese Medicine (TCM). Since ancient times, numerous Chinese scholars have experimented and attempted to directly observe and record the flow of Qi through various spiritual technologies, in order to come to a basic understanding of how it flows through our body; what is its role and function; how it connects us to nature, and indeed the whole universe etc.

The crux of TCM's finding is that Qi has profoundly healing properties.

The Core Concept of Qi

The three core concepts in TCM are Qi, yin and yang. A given amount of Qi is necessarily required by our body to maintain the delicate Yin and Yang balance, or the outcome can be disharmony.

When an individual's qi is balanced and in harmony, he keeps good health, is optimistic, cheerful and contended. When one's Qi is deficient, the outcome can be pain, sickness, suffering, and illness may occur.

- Qi is the source of all movement of the body: ascending, descending, entering and leaving
- Qi protects the body against external and internal pathological factors
- Qi regulates the production and flow of all body fluids - blood, tears, sweat, and urine
- Qi governs the functioning of all organs
- Qi regulates body temperature and keeps it warm

What Determines Qi?

Qi is acquired at birth and retained until the death of the organism. TCM practitioners insist that it has to be 'earned' throughout life and that implies that we have to look after it, otherwise we can lose this vital resource, and with it our physical and mental health.

The optimum flow of Qi in the body depends upon various lifestyle factors, such as the food we eat, exercise, our emotions, and exposure to environmental pollutants. It's also partially inherited from our parents from the time of the birth, and it shapes our appearance, thoughts, temperament, personality, body constitution and most importantly, our vulnerability to various diseases.

Qi or Chi Depletion

There are a variety of physical and emotional factors that can diminish a person's qi. Among the most common factors is stress and sleep deprivation. It could also be related to food choices, anxiety about shelter, the quality of water or air we breathe in, etc. In short, Qi is impacted by all the factors that hamper the proper functioning of our body.

On a very different plane, Qi can also deplete if there is a lack of mental stimulation, social interaction, and love. All these factors in isolation or together, can raise the level of the stress hormone in our body, which is called cortisol, which can impair the immune function and increase the risk of catching disease, cause depression and burnout. The final outcome could be the flow out of Qi from the body.

Signs and Symptoms of Qi Deficiency Can Include

- Thyroid disorders
- Irregular menstruation
- Infertility
- Anxiety
- Fatigue
- Autoimmune disorders
- Higher susceptibility to infections
- Muscular pains
- Allergies
- Chronic liver disease
- Abrupt changes in appetite and weight

How Can Qi Deficiency Be Treated?

Treatment will depend on the type of Qi deficiency, how long it's existed, and what's caused it. Blood investigation may be needed to determine the causes, some of which are better addressed by conventional medicine or addressed in conjunction with it.

Treatments may include:

✓ Nutritional therapies
✓ Use of Chinese herbs
✓ Major lifestyle adjustments

The Leaking of Qi

Leaking Qi, the body's inability to consolidate and hold in any type of fluid substance in the body. Leaking Qi can be caused by different conditions.

Imbalances in the 'Triple Heater' system are one specific cause that can alter fluid retention in the body that is essential for sustenance.

Excessive sweating can also lead to loss of essential fluids from the body leading to weakness in the Upper and Middle Jiao. This happens when the Qi of the lungs is too weak to control the skin function properly. If left untreated, that condition can dehydrate the skin and accelerate aging.

Qi Stagnation

When Qi doesn't flow smoothly, the outcome is discomfort.

In the early stages of qi disturbance, you may not notice or report the symptoms as they might be very weak or mild, but as your condition aggravates, the irritation and feeling of discomfort would become chronic.

TCM practitioners believe that stagnant Qi can manifest itself as rebellious Qi and appear in the form of coughing or nausea, with a loss of appetite.

Alternatively, stagnant qi may start to spread to other parts of the body, causing acidity, and digestive disorders. When acute, stagnant Qi can take the form of a heart attack.

Since Qi is nothing but energy, often stagnant Qi can transform into heat or Ascending Qi. Prolonged stress or anxiety can make this condition worse. The process can be arrested and reversed in the early stages, if the cause is properly identified and the source of stress is removed from the patient's environment. Later, when symptoms have moved from acute to chronic, even this measure may not yield adequate relief.

Building and Healing Chi

Nature has given everybody the restorative powers to build and gather the lost or depleted Qi. Since, Qi is a universal energy given to all, it can be gathered easily from our environment, but this calls for discipline and daily practice.

In TCM, the concept of Qi, as explained in the beginning of this Chapter, extends beyond the physical body, to even cover the mental and spiritual faculties. In mature, evolved, creative human beings, such as scholars, scientists and artists and spiritual leaders, Qi is perfectly balanced and it reflects at all levels—art, business, in their relationships, leadership styles, and child rearing practices.

Spiritual chi makes it possible for ordinary mortals to self-actualize their highest potential. It transcends them into higher realms of consciousness, which lie at the core of any religious experience or spiritual awakening.

Qigong, tai chi and other form of Taoist martial and healing arts assist in tapping into the inner reservoir of this chi-energy, and you can actually feel it coursing through your body.

To remain pain-free and in optimal health condition, the Qi must circulate freely and unobtrusively through the entire body, without disruption, in a smooth, powerful and purposeful manner.

The classic Chinese medical phrase for this kind of a flow is *teng jr bu tong*. If the circulation of your chi is blocked (*bu tong*), the straight outcomes are pain and disease (*teng*). Conversely, if the Qi in a person's acupuncture meridian lines are fully connected and circulating without blockages (*tong),* the person will experience neither pain, nor disease (*bu tong*) - *tong jr bu teng.*

This is the basic goal of TCM that can be achieved through acupressure, acupuncture, tai chi, qigong and other forms of martial arts. Balancing and connecting you to your Qi, so there are no blockages and you can get rid of all kinds of pain, disease and anxiety to live your life to the fullest.

Qi or Chi Activating

The first step to start healing yourself is to believe that you are not lacking in Qi. You can be your own healer. You were meant to be your healer. You have that resource within you.

The protective layer shielding you may have thinned out without nutrition, care and depressive circumstances, but this Qi is always available to you for the asking. You can awaken it anytime with the practice of deep breathing, meditation and exercise. Inculcate positive habits and thoughts inside you. Surround yourself with green beautiful environment as much as you can. All this self-work and activation will keep Qi in balance both internally and externally and rest assured that you will be completely healed.

Physical Activities to Activate Your Qi

In order to re-activate your Qi naturally and replenish your cells and improve the circulation of energy throughout your body, a very simple exercise would be to rub your hands and palms vigorously every morning when you get up.

Next rub your knuckles and your nails for a few minutes each. Then, shake your hands down by your side vigorously for a few minutes and proceed on to activate some of your pressure points. Please consult the meridian maps for instructions.

Take a couple of deep breaths and feel—actually feel – the Qi coursing freely through every nook and cranny of your body. Pat your neck, shoulders, inner, outer arms and inner outer legs/stomach area. Take a few more deep breaths and tune into the Qi coursing through you. Feel one with it.

Last but not the least, feel yourself grounded. Take deep breaths and imagine you are a strong tree with roots going deep into the ground and visualize yourself inhaling all the positive energy around you. Next, exhale all the negative energy out.

This simple exercise repeated a few times, will help you tune in, and balance your Qi every day!

The Concept of Full Qi

Full Qi, I've come to believe is the state when you begin to wield absolute control over the movement of Qi. There is no leaking or stagnation and the pure energy flows freely through every, while part of your body – unrestrained, and unrestricted with no blockages of any kind, whatsoever.

Interestingly, when you have full Qi, you can easily build upon this energy reservoir to ascend to the highest level of awareness possible.

You can direct it, as per your wish, to whichever part of your body is sick or ailing and heal yourself.

Most important, I have come to believe through my many years of practice and observation that one can also move one's Qi beyond body and time. But since this subject is beyond the scope of this book, I will take it up at another opportunity.

Chapter 7

Healing By Reiki

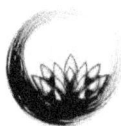

A woman got diagnosed with an abnormal growth in her uterus. Doctors ordered a slew of pathological tests - blood culture, biopsy, ultrasound and CT scan. The tests confirmed her worst fears – a malignant tumour that was growing too fast for comfort.

At twenty-eight with a six-year-old daughter, the news came as a bolt from the blue. She felt her fate was sealed and she slipped into acute clinical depression. That's when she found a Reiki master.

She gave her two short treatments of Reiki hands-on and also sent her Reiki, every night before going to bed. Alongside, the Reiki master asked her circle to pray for this young woman for almost a month.

A month later, when she went for a repeat ultrasound, before the planned surgery, there was no sign of the tumour! It had simply vanished, leaving no trace.

This may seem incredible, but it's true. I've personally experience and heard many such tales of miraculous recovery from my friends and acquaintances, who are deeply into this practice and have experienced its benefits.

What is Reiki?

Reiki is a spiritual healing art with its roots in ancient Japanese culture, dating back to the late 1800s. With Reiki it's possible to transfer the powerful universal energy from the practitioner's palms to a receptive patient.

Reiki can also be used for self-healing, as a supportive therapy, in conjunction with traditional medical care.

The form of Reiki that many people practice today, Usui Reiki, has been in use for over one hundred years.

History and Origin

The word Reiki originates from the Japanese root word (Rei) which means "Universal Life" and (Ki) which means "Energy". It's simply an effective channelizing of pure, spiritually guided energy to the sick and infirm for numerous health benefits.

Experts believe that the Reiki format that is currently in use was first developed in 1922 by a Japanese Buddhist scholar called Mikao Usui, who subsequently taught 2,000 people the technique during his lifetime. The practice become so popular that it soon began to spread to other, remote parts of the world, the U.S. in the 1940s, and then to Europe in the 1980s.

How It the Energy Transmitted?

Referred to as palm healing or hands-on healing, to administer Reiki, a practitioner uses his hands to transmit energy to another, and specifically to the diseased part of the receiver's body. Other than physical ailments (chronic or acute), Reiki healing can also be used to diffuse stress, anxiety, pain, loneliness, sadness, confusion, etc. — when a Reiki healer attempts to clear the pathways for the clogged energy in the recipient's body, using his hands as the instrument.

How Does Reiki Work?

We are alive and kicking today because we have this life force, prana or Qi coursing through us. This energy flows though definite pathways called chakras, meridians or nadis. It also creates an invisible field of energy, around us called the aura.

In Reiki it's believed that this life force also begins to deplete when we advertently or inadvertently begin to harbor negative thoughts or feelings about ourselves. Such thoughts conflict with the life force and cause disruption in its flow. Reiki restores the energy back into the affected organ. It clears, straightens and heals the blocked energy pathways, thus restoring the person to health the natural way.

If nothing, it induces deep relaxation, help people cope with real or imagined challenges, removes anxiety and instills an overall sense of well-being. Reiki recipients describe it as "immensely healing."

Levels of Reiki Treatment

Typically, there are three (sometimes four) levels that can be attained in Reiki practice, through consistent and persistent study, discipline and practice.

Reiki Initiation

There is a special ceremony that marks the elevation of a Reiki practitioner from one level to the next, which is called Reiju (Ray-joo) in Japanese. Reiju is performed by the Reiki Master, who opens and expands the main energy channels of the student's body, thus allowing the universal life force to permeate the student's body.

This ceremony marks powerful energy exchange from the master to the student, before which the student has to undergo a period of intense practice and self-watch, allowing no negative thought to vitiate his immediate environment.

Here is a breakdown of the three levels of Reiki:

LEVEL ONE : The First Degree

Some people are naturally gifted to be healers. They get drawn to Reiki practice like magnets. Others consider it as an instrument for self-realization, and actualization of their spiritual awakening. Whatever be the motive, this level consists of four attunements or what are called 'energy activations' over a two-day span.

The four attunements given in Level One open up the physical body to a sort of a Reiki experience, when he is ready to absorb the healing energy within himself and effectively channel it to others, as well.

At this level the maximum positive impact of the energy exchange is felt on the physical body. This level of Reiki attunement can be very powerful in curing chronic diseases in the person receiving the attunement. The physical changes can be observed within days following the attunement.

In the interim, the native's body adjusts to the Reiki energy and at times, the person may feel a sense of dizziness, empty, or have vivid dreams—all of which are signs of detoxification, so should not worry the person. As more Qi enters your body and creates a new energetic field, the physical and etheric bodies will start to be cleared of denser patterns that do not belong to your person.

LEVEL TWO : Second Degree

This is the next, logical step that also involves some degree of spiritual development. At this stage, as a willing channel of Reiki energy, you are actually making a commitment to yourself that you will attempt to go past your physical boundaries.

Once you allow yourself to open to this all-pervasive, all-powerful Universal Life Energy, there would be no turning back. At Level Two, your energy reservoir that you can subsequently share with others expands manifold, as you are able to tap into the energy source that is running through the entire cosmos.

While Level One attunement kept you bound to the physical plane, the Level Two attunements will take you on a higher emotional and mental plane, where you will experience the transforming powers of the Life Energy, even more strongly.

This Reiki Level Two is distant or across time-space, where you can begin working with someone who is not physically present, but still connected to you on a mental plane.

At Level Two, you become supremely aware of the three Reiki symbols or keys that you can use in your practice for long-distance, remote healing. The keys can effectively be used in direct sessions also to unlock the healing potential of another person to whom you are passing on the Reiki energy.

LEVEL THREE : Third Degree

Level three is the final level of training in Reiki practice. At this level, Reiki masters teach Heart Attunement so that can begin to treat others. At this stage, the student metamorphoses into a Reiki Master.

The tradition is that when a practitioner receives the Master attunement, they have received the highest degree of self-realization and has become the perfect channel for Reiki practice.

Chapter 8

Yoga – Asanas and Mudras

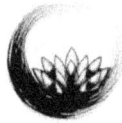

Sangeeta Kapoor, aged 28 suffered from chronic symptoms of Rheumatoid Arthritis, i.e. severe joint pain and stiffness. She found it difficult to carry out even everyday chores such as brushing her teeth or combing her hair, without help. For someone like Sangeeta, whose passion was daily, brisk walking, rheumatoid arthritis was crushing and deeply depressing. It put brakes on her once active life.

To improve her mobility, she underwent a partial hip replacement surgery in 2010. However her body didn't react well to the metal implant, which only increased her pain. She had to undergo a second surgery to set right things, but when that too didn't help, she started to practice yoga.

The heat and fluidity that yoga brought with it, helped ease the pain in her joints, making her regain more and more of her confidence with each class she attended. After a couple of weeks of attending regular yoga sessions, Sangeeta could even attempt complicated yoga asanas, such as headstand in the center of a room. No disease, Karen determined, could rob her of healthy living.

People in India have been practicing and perfecting yoga for thousands of years. Yoga Sutra of Patanjali, the sacred text of 200 AD delves deep into the foundations of the yoga philosophy. It also describes the inner workings of the human mind, providing an eight-step method that can help control restlessness and lead to lasting peace.

The eight limbed path or the Ashtanga yoga, which is the core of Patanjali's Yoga Sutra gives a structural framework for the practice of yoga. One who practices all these eight limbs of the path manages to achieve a perfect balance of various elements. By making practitioners feel absolutely complete within themselves, yoga helps them experience intimate connectivity with the divine.

The word "Asana" in Sanskrit stands for a physical posture. In general terms it is a specific position that you can hold comfortably for a longer period of time. When Patanjali wrote the Yoga Sutras in the 2nd century BC, he defined the meditation posture as "Asana." The physical postures were termed as "Yoga Vyayam." Nevertheless, with time, all dynamic Yoga exercises started being known as Asanas.

It is from the natural positions and movements of animals that most asanas are derived from. These poses even carry the names of the animals such as "deer," "tiger," "cat," and "hare." These positions and movements come with their own set of natural benefits, which is why animals use them instinctively. The effects can be seen through regular practice of yoga.

For instance, you can release your aggression and emotions by practicing Bhujangasana (The Cobra). Marjari or the cat is good for stretching your body and spine. Shashankasana (The Hare) can be great for relaxation.

Asanas can not only improve the functioning of your cardiovascular system, nervous system, and the lymphatic system, they can also be beneficial for your muscles, joints, mind, psyche, as well as the Chakras (energy centers). Being psychosomatic exercises, they tend to strengthen and balance your entire nervous system, thereby stabilizing and harmonizing your state of mind. With practice of these exercises, you will start experiencing a sense of contentment, relaxation, peace, inner freedom, and amazing clarity of mind. Correct performance of yoga exercises depends on how relaxed you are physically and mentally. This is when you get to experience maximum benefits of these asanas.

Every movement has to be coordinated with your breath, to make your Yoga practice more harmonious. With the deepening of every breath (which happens on its own accord), your body's metabolism and circulation get stimulated. Every time you exhale, you need to focus on relaxing the muscles in the tense areas of your body.

Asana, as per Patanjali's Yoga Sutra, is a steady and a comfortable posture. It doesn't refer to any specific pose; but only suggests that it is a steady and comfortable position one should seek for, while practicing.

Different asanas have been described historically by texts and teachers. In fact as per the classic texts of Hatha Yoga, there are about 84 asanas that were taught by Lord Shiva. The first four of these, namely Siddhasana, Padmasana, Bhadrasana and Simhasana, are considered crucial for achieving spiritual perfection.

The Importance of Asanas

The asanas are best practiced on an empty stomach. No excessive pressure or force is to be used while practicing them. If you want to enhance the benefits of the poses that you practice, you can think of combining your asanas with your pranayama practice. While doing so, your mind has to be aware and your focus has to be on uniting your body with your mind and your breathing. There are specific asanas that work well in alleviating certain health problems and physical issues.

Benefits of Practicing Asanas:
✓ It increases strength and flexibility
✓ It removes blocks if any along the pathways of energy
✓ It helps in synchronizing the body and mind
✓ It stimulates each and every physiological system of the body including the digestive, circulatory and the immune systems.
✓ It helps develop the focus and the mindfulness that is crucial for practicing meditation
✓ It stimulates the energy in the body, opening up the nadis and the chakras

The aim of practicing various asanas is to feel your body and make it stronger for performing pranayamas. As pranayama exercise is directly connected with 'prana' energy, and the objective is to release this energy during a pranayama session, if your body is weak or unhealthy, it won't be able to absorb that much energy and the exercise may in fact turn out to be counterproductive for that person, both physically and emotionally. That is specifically the reason why a person who is weak, sick or swollen, should be advised not to do pranayama.

The Most Important Asanas

Since a description of each asana is beyond the scope of this book, we will describe only the most significant ones in this section.

Suryanamaskar or Sun Salutation

Without the sun there can be no life on earth. An ancient method of paying respect or showing gratitude to this source of all life forms on earth, is called Surya Namaskar or Sun Salutation. It is a set of 12 postures that represent a complete body work out. Performed 12 times within a time span of 12 to 15 minutes, this exercise is equivalent to performing 288 powerful Yoga Asanas. It is an excellent blend of warming-up poses as well as the intense Yoga Asanas.

As per the ancient yogis, every part of our body is governed by a specific deva or divine impulse of light. The solar plexus that is located behind the navel is the one that is connected to and controlled by the Sun. By practicing Surya Namaskar regularly, we can enhance the size of this solar plexus, which in turn increases creativity, enhances intuitive abilities, improves decision-making and boosts confidence as well as leadership skills. Surya Namaskar can be done in the morning or evening, while facing the sun.

Vrikashana or the Tree Pose

Vriksh in Sanskrit means tree and Vrikshasana (pronounced as Vrik-Shah-Sana) is a yogic pose that resembles the tree. While improving your focus and concentration this Asana helps increase your body's balance. It is best performed early in the morning on an empty stomach.

Viparitakarani

Viparita in Sanskrit means reversed or inverted and *karani* means making or doing. So Viparitakarani is the act of inverting. The hatha yoga pradipika considers Viparitakarani as a mudra that directs the kundalini or vitality upwards within the body. The asanas on the other hand create steadiness.

As per some of the Hindu sacred texts, Viparita Karani reduces the appearance of wrinkles and keeps seniority under control, by enabling blood flow to all parts of the body. Any infirmity will be calmed by this asana.

Advantages of Viparita Karani

One of the postures considering best for healing and rejuvenation, Viparita Karani if practiced regularly, can improve each and every system of the body including digestion and circulation. The restorative version of this asana has the power to change an agitated mind into a clear and calm one. A few more benefits of practicing Viparita Karani include:

• Relief to cramped or worn out legs and feet
• Extension of the back of the neck, back of the legs, and the front of the middle
• Alleviation of gentle spinal pain
• A quiet and alleviated psyche

Halasana

An inverted yoga posture, Halasana is recommended for intermediate yoga practitioners. 'Hal' in Sanskrit means Plow which is a farming tool that is used for agriculture in India. In Halasana the shape of the body will resemble a plow.

A folded inversion posture that ranges between the intermediate and advanced levels, this asana is best practiced at the end of a Yoga session. Practiced astutely, halasana has the power to elevate the body to the state of *pratyahara* (the fifth stage of Patanjali's Ashtanga Yoga which is represented by the withdrawal of senses). This asana should ideally be followed by *shavasana* or a round of *pranayama*.

Benefits of Halasana

Halasana is said to rejuvenate the abdominal muscles, increase the suppleness of the spine and stimulate the female reproductive organs.

- It improves the strength and tone of the back muscles, the spinal cord, and the leg as well as the abdominal muscles.
- By increasing the pressure on the nerves in the neck region, it improves the efficiency of the spinal nerves and enhances the operation of the sympathetic nervous system.
- It stimulates the functioning of the thyroid, parathyroid, pituitary, and adrenal glands, which regulate all the other endocrinal glands, thereby improving the overall functioning of the endocrine system.
- It improves the blood circulation in the body
- It is useful in conditions such as bronchitis, asthma and dyspepsia
- It relaxes and stretches the muscle ligaments of the thighs and calves
- By improving the functioning digestive system, this asana helps those who are suffering from gastric problems and constipation.
- It normalizes the blood-glucose levels and benefits people who are diabetic
- By stimulating the reproductive organs, it helps women deal with their menopausal symptoms
- It strengthens the immune system and proves to be therapeutic for people suffering from headache, backache, insomnia, sinusitis, and infertility

Shavasana or the Corpse Pose

A restorative asana, s*avasana,* or *shavasana,* is a key component of yoga. *Shava* in Sanskrit refers to a Corpse, which is why this asana is also called the corpse pose. It is almost always practiced near the end of a yoga session or after *vinyasa*. However, it can also be practiced at the beginning of the practice to calm the body or in the middle of a

ちょっと

sequence for resting. If done at the end of the yoga session, savasana can be followed by seated meditation.

Shavasana is said to stimulate the *muladhara* (root) chakra, as it connects the entire length of the body with the earth. By energizing this chakra shavasana can ground an individual, providing him with the inner stability that he needs for his personal growth.

Benefits of Savasana

One of the most beneficial asanas, *savasana* can help in relieving mild depression, insomnia, high blood pressure, headaches, and fatigue. It promotes equanimity in the entire body, calming the nervous system completely. It relaxes the fatigued muscles, tensed shoulders and tightened jaws. As the eyes quieten down, the mind enters into a calm state.

Steps to Perform Shavasana or Corpse Pose:

- While lying on your back, rotate your legs in and out for a while and then rest them on your sides.
- Separate your arms from your body with your palms facing upwards.
- Give your body a complete stretch starting from your shoulders all the way to your feet.
- Take slow and deep breaths right from the abdomen.
- Be in this position for several minutes while focusing on your breathing
- When you are ready to get up, gently bend your knees, push yourself to one side and come to a sitting position.

Yoga Nidra

Yogic Sleep or Yoga Nidra is a form of pratyahara that lets you go deep into conscious relaxation. A preliminary and active form of meditation, this helps you reap most of the benefits of meditation.

In this state your body is asleep but you will be in a state of complete awareness. Your mind will not drift into dreams or wander aimlessly. The "witness" in you emerges while you are in this state. This is the part of your Self that watches your experience, without being attached to it. An unemotional state with absence of thoughts, this state brings into you, a lot of joy and peace. Rather than a technique, Yoga Nidra is best termed as a state of consciousness.

How to Achieve the State of Yoga Nidra?

In order to achieve the state of Yoga Nidra one will have to undergo a session of guided meditation, with a teacher giving instructions. Through his or her voice, the teacher guides the awareness of the student and helps the student go deeper within himself. The first focal point in this state is the voice of the teacher.

The teacher starts by instructing the student to examine individual parts of his body and seek out areas that are tensed. The pranic flow in these areas will be disturbed. By following the guidance of the teacher, the student attempts to relax these areas, thus making the prana flow freely. Throughout the session the teacher's voice will guide the student. So if the teacher's voice is the first focal point, the second one is each body part. By the end of the session, the entire body of the student would be deeply relaxed. All through the session the student is completely awake, which is why Yoga Nidra is called the state of consciousness.

The Origin of Yoga Nidra

The term Yoga Nidra is quite ancient and no one knows where it originated from. However it is mentioned in a few scriptures such as Devi Bhagavata (when Lord Vishnu manifests creation reclining on Naga Shesha), Taravali, and Hatha Yoga. Nevertheless, the concept is not explained in any of these references.

Benefits of Yoga Nidra

An extraordinary technique, Yoga Nidra helps in self-healing as well as developing consciousness. Once in the deepest states of relaxation, the body's physiology achieves a state of perfect balance, which in turn causes the healing.

- Yoga Nidra works on all the systems of the body such as the nervous system, the immune system, and the endocrine system, as well as on the organs of the body.
- When used along with the treatments for diseases such as cancer, heart disease, chronic fatigue, pain, and autoimmune disorders, it can work like an outstanding complementary approach, supporting the process of healing.
- It increases self-awareness and lets a practitioner learn everything there is to know about himself.

Savasana vs Yoga Nidra

More often than not, people tend to confuse Yoga Nidra with Savasana. In Savasana you just lie still on your back in deep meditative relaxation. Nevertheless, Yoga Nidra captures your attention in a much more dynamic way. It is a guided relaxation session wherein instructions from a teacher guide your awareness throughout your body in a calm yet brisk pace. It triggers deep relaxation. If you get lost in your thoughts and tend to forget what you are doing, you only have to listen to the instructions to get back on the track. This way Yoga Nidra helps even the beginners in entering a state of deep relaxation. Having prior experience with Yoga Nidra can help you appreciate Savasana in its true sense.

Yog Mudras and How Are These Different from Yoga Asanas

'*Mudra*' in Sanskrit means 'gesture'. Yoga Mudras are gestures that are used to heal different parts of the body, by focusing on the energy in them. Yoga Mudras are generally practiced during mediation. They are also incorporated with pranayama or deep breathing. Most mudras are performed using hands; but there is one mudra called the Kechari Mudra which is done using the tongue.

Mudras can be performed at any time. However, healing can be more effective if they are performed sitting in the lotus position. Not only can mudras be used to heal certain ailments, they can also be used as a prevention measure, contributing to the overall health. Through continuous practice of mudras, you can come across minute changes in your body that can trigger healing processes corresponding to different body parts.

Hasta Mudra (Hand Mudra)

Hasta in Sanskrit refers to the hand. Hasta Mudra refers to a hand gesture which can be symbolic, ritualistic or even therapeutic. You can practice hasta mudras while standing, sitting or walking, as long as your body is relaxed and the posture, symmetrical. In asana practice hasta mudras help in directing the flow of energy and in meditation they help in focusing your mind.

Apart from this, hasta mudras can also be used to stimulate different emotions and spiritual reactions within the body. You can stimulate the reflexes from your hand to the brain just by touching, pointing, curling, or pressing together different fingers or parts of your hands in various ways.

The Philosophy of Mudra Therapy

The benefits of Mudra therapy confirm the fact that your health is literally in your hands. The five fingers of your hand represent the *Panchamahabhootas* or the five major building blocks the entire universe is made up of - Sky (Ether), Air, Fire, Water and Earth.

- The Thumb represents Fire or Agni
- The Index finger represents Air or Vayu
- The Middle Finger represents the Ether or Aakash (Sky)
- The Ring finger represents the earth or Prithvi
- The Small finger represents Water or Jala

Any imbalance in any of these five elements can emerge in the form of a disease. You can try a few Hasta Mudras to achieve a perfect balance of these five elements.

Three Important Yog Mudras

There are many types of mudras that can be used for different purposes. Here are three basic types of mudras that can help heal diseases and improve the overall wellbeing:

Gyan Mudra

Also known as Vayu Vardhak Mudra, this is one mudra that is popularly recognized all over the world. By exciting the root chakra this mudra helps in reducing tension, stress and depression. Not only does this calm the mind, it also leads to spiritual awakening.

Since it stimulates the air element of the body, the gyan mudra is said to increase the memory power, improve the functioning of the nervous system, and enhance the production of the pituitary gland production. Apart from improving the focus, it also helps in sharpening the brain and building mental power. Done regularly, it can be used to treat many kinds of mental and psychological disorders including stress, anger, depression, anxiety and insomnia.

How to Perform the Gyan Mudra?

With your palms facing upward, touch the tip of your index finger to the tip of your thumb. The other three fingers should be straight. You can perform this pose early in the morning for about 35 to 40 minutes at a stretch. Alternatively you can also perform this in three sessions of 10 to 15 minutes each, any time during the day.

Prana Mudra

Prana in Sanskrit means life and Prana Mudra increases the pranic energy (vitality) within your body. By boosting your energy levels, it improves your eyesight, reduces vitamin deficiencies, removes exhaustion, and increases your body's resistance to diseases. Practiced while fasting, it can reduce your hunger pangs, giving you a good night's sleep. By stimulating and energizing the entire body, this mudra controls the movements of all your internal organs.

How to Perform the Praana Mudra?

Touch the tips of your ring finger and your little finger with the tip of your thumb. The other two fingers are to be kept straight. While doing this Mudra, take regular breaths for a few seconds, breathing in and out. Practice this Mudra for 30 to 40 minutes every day to see the results.

Aakash Mudra

Aakash Mudra is best practiced during dhyaan, when you are trying to connect with the divine. It can also help in getting rid of a lot of chronic health problems. Aakash Mudra is related to the space, or what is referred to as the ether element. Negative emotions, such as fear, anger, etc. get replaced by positive feelings and thoughts, with the regular practice of this mudra, and you feel rejuvenated and charged-up with energy.

How to Perform the Akash Mudra?

Touch the tip of your thumb to the tip of your middle finger. Try and keep the rest of the fingers in a comfortable position.

Chapter 9

Yoga – Breathing, Pranayama and Bandhas

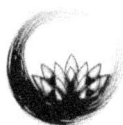

*A yogi measures the span of life by the number
of breaths, not by the number of years.*
— *Swami Sivananda*

Experts contend that by the simple act of breathing 15 times in a minute, we can hope to live to 75 or beyond. But if we breathe 10 times per minute, we can last for 100 years. The speed at which we breathe determines, or is directly proportionate to the longevity. In other words, faster we breathe, shorter our life. That's the reason dogs have shorter lives – no more than 12 years.

And that's the reason we are warned not to work up a fit, because anger quickens the pace of breathing and that takes away a few years from your life. By choosing to remain in an angry state you are doing no one any harm, except yourself.

Breathing in Yoga

A yoga teacher will constantly instruct his students to "breathe consciously" in the training session, do you know why?

Because breathing is a fundamental law in yoga. Breathing, nay correct breathing is what puts us in touch with the inner reservoir of energy, or the life force within us. By breath alone we are able to navigate different levels of consciousness, like a sailor astride choppy waters.

Further, breathing correctly has a decidedly conscious impact on our physical, mental and emotional states. It maintains the equilibrium. It keeps us grounded to the present. When a person is asked to concentrate on nothing but his breathing pattern – the inhalation and exhalation, that completes one cycle of breath – for that split second, we begin to live in the present, in the here and now. In this state, neither the past nor the future matters. We are grounded to nothing but the present.

This is why breathing consciously is a "little meditation" in its own right. However this is just the starting point. We will explore and examine this subject further as we dig deeper into this Chapter.

When we breathe correctly and consciously – aware of each inhalation and exhalation – we get to activate a different part of our brain. Unconscious or involuntary breathing is controlled by the medulla oblongata, which lies in the brain stem, the most primitive part of the human brain.

But conscious breathing is governed and regulated by a more advanced section of our brain, which is the cerebral cortex. Conscious breath activates this section of the brain. It sends a powerful nerve impulse from the cortex to the portion of the human brain that controls emotions. That is why, stimulating the cerebral cortex has an immediate, beneficial impact on our emotional state. We feel immensely relaxed. In short, through conscious breathing, we are able to wield complete control over our emotional state. By a simple switch from medulla oblongata to the cerebral cortex, we are able to choose, whether to be happy and relaxed. Or worried or tense. The choice is ours.

The technique is extremely simple. The cerebral cortex gets stimulated by the simple act of the exhalation process – when you gradually and watchfully release your breath. At this point of time, the cerebral cortex sends inhibitory impulses to the respiratory center of our midbrain. These inhibitory impulses from the cerebral cortex get transmitted to an area of the hypothalamus, which is concerned with emotions, and the feeling is of release of tension and relaxation.

Full Yogic Breath or Pranayama

The term is derived from the Sanskrit root word, prana, meaning the "life force," and *ayama*, meaning an "extension" of this life force.

Pranayama is a set of breathing exercises taught in yoga practice, benefits all three doshas (fault lines) - vata, pitta, and kapha – which is one of the most important tenet in Ayurveda, the most important treatise on ancient Hindu practice of medicine.

Pranayama revitalizes the entire body, in particular the vital organs, which get worn down by disease, infection, worry and other cares of earthy life. Daily practice of pranayama relieves stress, activates a dull mind, stimulates our parasympathetic nervous system, and induces a calmer state in the individual.

There is no prescribed, set time to do pranayama, but it's been observed to be most beneficial when done intensely for at least five to fifteen minutes every day—preferably on an empty stomach, early in the morning.

The Four Stages of Pranayama

- **Puraka** (Inhalation) - The steady drawing in of air and filling the lungs with oxygen.
- **Abhyantara Kumbhaka** (Pausing after the inhalation) - The intentional cessation of inhalation, as you hold your breath inside you.
- **Rechaka** (Exhalation) - Release of the breath in a steady, conscious movement. Returning the lungs to their formal, relaxed state.
- **Bahya Kumbhaka** (Pausing after the exhalation) - A state of calm awareness preceding the next inhalation. A moment of quiet reflection. Just being in the present.

Each of these four stages of pranayama has the effect of enhancing your total awareness. It's an important tool for deep introspection and ultimate enlightenment.

Whenever you have the time and feel depleted of energy, practice Full Yogic Breath in the following simple steps:

Deeply inhale air into your body from your lower abdomen. When you feel that your abdomen is full, continue inhalation to fill your mid torso and once that is full, fill your upper chest and lungs.

In the same manner, release your breath gradually, first from the upper chest, then the mid torso and finally the lower abdomen, without any pause between the two breaths.

Repeat the cycle a few times.

Anulom Vilom/Alternate Nostril Breathing/ Nadi Shodhana

This exercise purifies the nadis, which as we discussed in the Chapter on the Chakras are the nodes or the energy channels in our astral body. Regular practice of Anulom Vilom calms the mind. It oxygenates the blood, and effectively transmits oxygen to the deeper level of cells, tissues and organs thereby flushing out all the harmful, disease-causing toxins from our body.

Practitioners follow a daily routine of pranayama as an isolated technique, or weave it into their daily hatha yoga practice.

How to Do Anulom Vilom?

The basic technique is to breathe alternatively through each nostril, while the other is held closed with the fingers. The thumb finger is used to hold the right nostril, while the person breathes normally through the left; and the ring finger is used to hold the left nostril shut.

To begin, follow these steps:

- Sit on a mat, cross-legged, shut your eyes and keep your spine straight.
- Shut your right nostril with your right thumb and begin to inhale slowly through your left nostril. Take in as much air as you can in each breath, till your lungs are full.
- Now remove your thumb from the right nostril and exhale from the right while holding your left nostril shut.

> **About Pranayama**
>
> Through Pranayama, or breath control, it's possible to both energize and relax our bodies. Pranayama gives two-fold benefits – it cures diseases and it also relaxes the mind for meditation.

- Now, inhale through your right nostril and shut your right nostril, while exhaling from the left nostril.
- Repeat this procedure for at least ten to fifteen times to derive full benefits from this exercise. Don't overstrain yourself.

The Appropriate Ratio

Beginners can start in the ratio of 1:1 for inhalation and exhalation. This implies, you inhale for four seconds through one nostril then exhale from the other nostril in the next four seconds. With slow and regular practice, the ratio can be altered to 1:2, where the inhalation lasts for four seconds, and exhalation for eight seconds.

Benefits of Anuloma Viloma

You will begin to feel positive vibes in your body, besides:

- Increased oxygen supply to the brain, leading to a state of calm and relaxation.
- It improves blood circulation.
- Corrects heart-related problems.
- Improves focus and concentration.
- Prevents lifestyle-related diseases, such as blood pressure and diabetes.
- Very effective in treating constipation, acidity, allergies of all kinds. Even corrects snoring, provides relief to asthmatic patients, relieves headaches, neurological issues, and heart-related ailments and clears depression.
- Removes blockage of the blood vessels.
- Controls obesity.

The Three Bandhas and Their Meaning

Literally translated, it means to lock, hold, retain or tighten a position in order to direct prana (life force) to a particular area of the body. While in yoga, the emphasis is on keeping a still pose, in bandha one has to hold that asana (position) for a longer duration. While scholars study bandhas in context to pranayama, but they also have their own individual, beneficial effects.

Mula Bandha

Emerging from the Sanskrit word *mula,* meaning "root" or "base," mula refers to the base of the torso and it is related to the *muladhara,* or the root chakra. Energizing this chakra is believed to ground the individual and provide inner stability for personal growth. The purpose of the mula bandha is to prevent energy from flowing out of the body, instead drawing and directing it inwards through the spinal cord and the chakras.

Practice

✓ Inhale deeply and hold your breath.
✓ Place your hands on the knees, raise the shoulders and tilt the upper body forward.
✓ Concentrate on your Muladhara Chakra and firmly contract the anal muscles. Hold the muscular contraction and the breath as long as possible and comfortable.
✓ Then exhale gradually, and return to the normal position.
✓ Breathe normal.

Benefits

This exercise gives strength to the pelvic muscles, and provides relief from hemorrhoids and congestion in the pelvic region of the body. It is also known to have a calming effect on the autonomic nervous system. On the spiritual plane, this bandha activates the Muladhara Chakra, and awakens Kundalini Shakti.

Caution: Because of its intensive nature, Mula Bandha should be practiced only under the guidance of an expert.

Sanskrit Shloka

Apanpranayoraikyam kshayo mutrapurishayoh |
Yuva bhavati vrudhopi satatam mulbandhanat

Meaning

Apanvayu, as mentioned before is the downward flow of energy. With deliberate contraction, apanvayu gets lifted upwards. This is the main purpose of the mula bandha. The regular study of mula bandha results in merging apan and prana. A straight outcome of practicing this exercise is that excretions get minimized and even an older person begins to feel young and rejuvenated.

Uddiyana Bandha – Lifting the Diaphragm

The second bandha is Uddiyana. In Sanskrit, it means to fly or rise up. In this lock position, imagine that all your insides are flying upwards, which includes your diaphragm, stomach, and abdominal organs.

The Steps

- Sit upright.
- Inhale deeply.
- Then exhale slowly, while trying to move your stomach muscles to the inside.
- Next, lift your ribs a little and try and pull the muscles in the upward direction. You will feel the diaphragm being pushed up.
- Try to hold this position briefly, when the breath is fully exhaled.
- When there is an urgent need to inhale, the bandh must be released gradually.

Note: The muscles of the stomach must be totally relaxed and feel flexible to be able to do this exercise.

The Benefits

This bandh opens up blockages in the Manipura Chakra for the benefit of the heart and lungs. Additionally, it activates the intestinal area, relieves constipation and directs energy up the central channel from the earth, water, and fire centers into the heart chakra. It stimulates the pancreas and prevents diabetes. It also tones the abdomen, strengthens the diaphragm, stimulates gastric juices, aids digestion, and rids the digestive tract of various toxins. Lastly, it strengthens our immune system and calms the mind, while making it stress-free.

Caution: Do not practice this Bandha if you are a patient of high blood pressure. Women who are menstruating or pregnant should not practice this bandha. Also, don't practice it if you are suffering from stomach ache or have any kind of heart trouble. Refrain from practicing this bandh if you are suffering from diseases like hernia, stomach or intestinal ulcers etc.

Sanskrit Shloka

Nabherurdhwamadhaschapi tanam kuryatprayatnatah |
Shanmasbhyasenmrutyum jayatyeva na samshayah ||

Meaning

If a yogi practices this bandh consistently for six months, he or she can even win over death. A shloka after this promises that a regular practice of this bandh can also lead to mukti, which implies liberation or self-realization.

The Jalandhar Bandh

The name Jalandhara Bandha, or throat lock is derived from Sanskrit where jalan means 'net' and dhara means 'stream' or 'flow'. This exercise benefits the network of nadis (blood vessels and nerves) running through our neck region.

The throat locks holds the fluid flowing down to vishuddhi from bindu and prevents it from falling into the digestive fire. In this way prana is saved and not wasted.

The Technique

It involves simultaneously lowering the chin and lifting the sternum.

The Steps

- Sit in Padmasan or Siddhasan. Both are good positions to practice this bandh.
- Inhale deeply and hold your breath.
- Press the chin firmly against your chest.
- Concentrate on the Vishuddhi Chakra and hold the breath for as long as you possibly can, without discomfort.
- Raise your head and with a long exhalation return to the normal position.
- Breathing normally.
- Repeat the cycle at least five times.

Benefits – This exercise activates the inner energy reservoir, especially the Vishuddhi Chakra.It develops concentration power and is good for prevention of throat diseases and for regulating thyroid function. This bandh also helps circulatory and respiratory systems, balances thyroid metabolism and is good for mental relaxation. Additionally, it regulates the flow of blood and prana to the heart, head and the endocrine glands in the neck (thyroid and para-thyroid).On the spiritual plane, the bandha presses the Ida and Pingala channels and allows the prana to pass through sushumna.

Precautions – This bandh is not recommended for natives suffering from respirational problems or high or low blood pressure. Those with stiff necks and spondylitis should also abstain. Hold the locked posture by lifting the chest rather than by pressing it down with the chin. This will relax your throat muscles and your breathing will return to normal. Never force your chin to your sternum.

Sanskrit Shloka

Kanthasankochanam krutva chibukam hridaye nyaset |
Jalandharakrute bandhe shodashadharbandhanam |
Jalandharam mahamudra mrityoeach kshayakarini ||

Meaning

The chin is to be pressed onto the heart after contracting the throat. Jalandhar Bandh supports sixteen types of bandhas and counters disease and death.

Breathing with Mula Bandha

This is an important technique that I have practiced and refined, so follow it carefully.

Contract your pelvic muscles. Inhale and then exhale while gradually relaxing your body. No need to hold your breath. Repeat as per your comfort level. This technique will not just increase your energy level manifold but also prevent energy leak from your body and keep your aura intact.

Chapter 10

All About Meditation

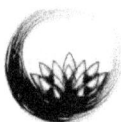

Contrary to popular belief, there is nothing religious about meditation. It is only a momentary pause of thoughts. It is like holding your breath under water or a stop you take while walking at a rapid pace. It is like the vacation you take when you are between jobs.

Innately human, meditation comes very naturally and easily to us. Try sitting under a tree next to a river and focus on the sound of the water. You may experience a time when your thoughts have paused naturally even if it is for just a few minutes. This is when your mind is at peace. Rest comes naturally to the mind when you are watching something that is calming – like the magnificence of the stars that emerge in the sky as the world grows darker and quieter.

This kind of rest that the mind gets is healing for the body. It helps in rebuilding the brain tissues and prevents many psychological disorders such as ADD and Alzheimer's. But no individual, organization, or for that matter even religion can own this inner peace. It is an experience – a state of being that individuals can access within themselves.

Among the eight components of Patanjali's Ashtanga Yoga, the sixth one is dharana or concentration. Dhyana or meditation is the seventh limb and Samadhi, or enlightenment, the final limb. Samadhi is the state where the meditating person merges with the very object of meditation. It is the ultimate bliss that an individual can ever experience. The last three limbs of Patanjali's ashtanga yoga are collectively known as antar atma sadhana (innermost quest) and are often studied together.

Trataka on Candle

Hatha Yoga Pradipika, the traditional text on the practices of Hatha Yoga, talks about six cleaning techniques, one of which is Trataka. To practice this, you have to focus your gaze on a small point and look at it intently and unwaveringly until your eyes begin to tear. The object that you gaze upon can be internal or external. For instance, a flame of a candle would be an external object but something like the third eye would be an internal object. However, gazing at a candle flame happens to be the most commonly practiced form of Trataka.

Trataka Technique

- Place a candle on a small table and light it.
- Take a seat about 3 to 4 feet behind the small table with the candle, facing it. Make sure you are comfortable with your spine upright and shoulders and arms totally relaxed. It would be great if you can assume a meditative posture without any movement for as long as you practice Trataka.
- The flame should be at your eye level and should remain steady throughout the concentration routine. Close the doors and windows, turn off the fan or air-conditioner and make sure there is no breeze that can disturb the flame.
- After taking a couple of deep breaths, close your eyes gently and focus on your breathing as you inhale and exhale. Do this for about five to seven breaths until your breath settles down.
- Look at the flame intently; making sure your gaze doesn't get distracted by any thoughts or external disturbances.
- Focus steadily on the flame, making sure you don't blink, for as long as possible. Stay still, avoiding any kind of body movements.

- Keep gazing at the flame until your eyes start watering. When you can't keep your eyes open anymore, close your eyes.
- You should be able to visualize an after-image of the flame once you close your eyes. Now bring this image at the center of your forehead, between your eyebrows (where your third eye is located).
- The clarity of this after image depends on the level and depth of your concentration.
- Once the image starts fading out, start focusing back on your breathing. Now watch the flow of your breath at the tip of your nose. Do this for about 7 to 8 breaths.
- At this point you can open your eyes. Repeat this entire gazing routine one more time.

Initially your eyes may start watering right after a few seconds. But with time, you should be able to gaze longer and extend your Trataka practice to about fifteen to twenty minutes.

Benefits of Trataka

As per the shloka 2.32 of Hatha Yoga Pradipika, Trataka is powerful enough to eradicate all eye diseases, sloth, and fatigue and prevents these problems from recurring. A few benefits of Trataka include:

- Better vision and improved eyesight
- Improved concentration, memory and intelligence
- More self-confidence, willpower and patience
- Calm mind with lots of inner peace and silence
- Greater clarity with improved decision making ability
- Freedom from mental, emotional and behavioral ailments
- Relief from stress
- Deep sleep with freedom from sleep-related disorders such as insomnia, nightmares, and headache

Trataka can make an excellent start for mantra meditation. As per Shloka 5.54 of Gherand Samhita, Trataka even promotes the perception of subtle manifestations which are referred to as clairvoyance.

A Few Important Meditation Techniques

i) **Symbolic Meditation with open eyes**
   Similar to Tratak, Symbolic Meditation is meditation practiced with open eyes. As you sit to meditate here you will have to focus on a symbol which could be a candle, a photo, a swastika or a cross. Make sure the symbol is kept at your eye level and the distance between your eyes and the symbol is not more than two feet. Concentrate on this symbol for as long as you are comfortable and then close your eyes and relax.

ii) **Symbolic meditation with closed eyes**
   Sit in meditation with closed eyes and picturize a symbol in your mind. It can be anything like a candle, a picture, or a symbol like swastika, Om or a cross. Now bring the focus to your third eye chakra, while still assuming the symbol. Do this for as long as you are comfortable. Unlike the above method, this one doesn't use any physical thing for concentration. It is only a copy of the symbol picturized with the help of the mind.

iii) **Closed eyes meditation without symbol**
   Although similar to the above method, this doesn't involve picturizing any symbol. You are only closing your eyes and concentrating on your third eye chakra. There is no symbol or anything. This type of meditation is very powerful.

iv) **Advanced meditation**
   Advanced meditation is more or less same as the closed eye meditation without symbol. You are closing your eyes and focusing on your third eye chakra. However, the concentration doesn't come from the inside of your body. It is from the outside of your body. Among all types of meditation, this is the one that is most powerful.

OM Chanting–Deep Silence is OM

In the Hindu mythology, Brahma was the only one who was there before the world came into existence. He was thinking how to become many from the one that he was. This thought led to a vibration that in turn settled into a sound of Om. The entire universe sprang into existence from this one vibration.

The vibration that comes from chanting Om matches the original vibrations that created the universe. Also known as Pranava, it is the sound of Om that runs through our breath, sustaining our lives. It represents the four states of a Supreme Being.

Being a diphthong (combination of two vowel sounds that lead to the sound of one vowel); O is usually pronounced as "AU" in Sanskrit. O is a diphthong and is usually spelled as AU in Sanskrit. While some say OM others call it AUM. The difference is only in their translation.

The sound Om was first mentioned in the Upanishads. The entire Mandukya Upanishad is dedicated to Om, regarding it as imperishable. As per this Upanishad, OM was there in the past, exists in the present, and will continue to be there in the future. Anything that exists beyond the bounds of time is referred to as Om.

The chanting of Om is not to be regarded as a religious practice. It refers to a cosmic sound, a universal syllable that led to the creation of the universe. It is the sacred sound of divine, a mysterious expression of eternity, timelessness, wisdom, and infinity. Om is at the core of our inner being; it is our higher self, our true nature. It is the first ever sound of creation and hence a holy monosyllable. It is life of all lives, the light of all lights, and the nectar of immortality. It is that eternal melody of peace, harmony, and love.

Symbolically embodying the divine energy or 'Shakti,' Om represents three main characteristics, namely Creation, Preservation, and Liberation. It is the universal energy that represents all languages.

Chapter 11

Everything About Your Central Nervous System

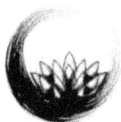

For every small action, every twitch of a muscle, every jerk of a limb, every breath we take, and every thought that crosses our mind, we use our Central Nervous System (CNS).

It is the system of the body that receives and processes all information from all other parts of the body. Comprising of a complex network of nerves and cells that carry messages to and from the brain and the spinal cord to various other parts of the body, the CNS is responsible for all cell-to-cell communication.

There are billions of nerve cells in the human body, perhaps not more than the number of stars in the Milky Way, but definitely more than the number of people on this planet.

The CMS has two parts – the central and the peripheral nervous system.

The central nervous system comprises of the brain and the spinal cord. The peripheral nervous system is made up of the somatic and the autonomic nervous systems. Both the brain and spinal cord are covered with a system of membranes, called meninges, surrounded by a cerebrospinal fluid. Because these are delicate organs, they are further protected by the bones of the skull and the vertebral column.

The peripheral nervous system is the connecting line between the brain/spinal cord and the rest of the organs. It has two parts somatic and autonomic. The somatic part of the peripheral nervous system, based on Greek word "soma" or body is responsible for transmitting both sensory information from the CNS and the five sense organs; as well as motor (related to movement) between CNS and the limbs – all with the help of a dense network of neurons.

The autonomic nervous system in contrast is responsible for regulating involuntary body functions, such as blood flow, heartbeat, digestion, and breathing. These functions are supposedly not in our voluntary (or wilful) control. This system is also divided in two functional parts - **The sympathetic system, which** regulates the primitive flight or fight response, when we perceive a dangerous situation; and the **parasympathetic system** that restores our body to normal functions once the perceived danger has passed.

When Many Sparks Unite...

The CNS is composed of a large numbers of excitable nerve cells and their tail ends, called neurons, which are supported by specialized tissue called neuroglia. These tail ends are called dendrites, axons or nerve fibres.

The interior of the CNS is organized into gray and white matter. Gray matter consists of nerve cells embedded in neuroglia and is of gray color. The white matter consists of nerve fibers embedded in neuroglia and is white colored due to the presence of lipid material in the myelin sheaths that cover the nerve fibers.

The neuron is the smallest unit of the CNS. Their special projections called dendrites bring information to the cell body and then take information away from the cell body. Neurons communicate with each other through an electrochemical process with the help of special connections called "synapses" and chemicals called "neurotransmitters" that are released at the synapse. It has been estimated that there are 1 quadrillion synapses in the human brain- 1,000,000,000,000,000 synapses!

Imagine that even as we sleep, our nervous system remains active— active enough to pick up and deliver impulses, from the environment and from each other.

The Primary Functions of CNS

The primary function of the central nervous system is communication, integration and co-ordination. The CNS receives information from all parts of the body in the form of stimuli and issues an appropriate response to this stimulus, in a meaningful manner.

For instance, when a person is walking, the CNS is receiving visual and integumentary cues – the texture of the surface he is walking on, its incline, the presence of obstacles, and so forth. If he is reading, the cues relate to the font size, the color, and also the context and the semantic meaning of the words.

Based on these stimuli, the CNS chooses an appropriate response. For instance in case of the walker, it commands the skeletal muscle to contract and expand to facilitate easy movement. We don't get to know about all these commands because once an infant has learnt to walk, all these movements are happening involuntarily, without conscious thought, as the CNS is already "programmed" like a computer.

A similar process of receiving complex stimuli and generating a co-ordinated response is required for all other motor and even cognitive (thought-related) activities – whether it is swimming, reading, striking up a conversation or mounting an immune response, against germs to fight disease.

All higher order mental functions, related to thought, retention and memory, speech and language learning are also controlled by the CNS. In language learning, the CNS learns to make sense of abstract symbols and sounds by associating them with concrete objects and emotions. Behavioral drivers such as motivation, ambition, reward and satisfaction are also mediated through the CNS. While, the primitive brain or the limbic system of the brain controls the expression of emotions and drives, such as pleasure, fear, anger, hunger, thirst, sleepiness and sexual desire.

In addition, involuntary reflexes – such as fear, fight and flight responses on perceiving a threat—are mediated by the spinal cord, thus providing protection and averting danger and injury to the self.

How the CNS Communicates – Chemical and Electrical Flashes

It's fascinating how neurons furiously work like little information-processing factories, continuously churning and tossing information about our internal and external environment, making sense of this glut of information, and coordinate responses appropriate to the situation and suitable to the person's current needs!

The Role of Nerve Impulses

A nerve impulse is the transmission of a coded signal from a stimulus along the membrane of the neuron. These are very much like electrical impulses. Nerve impulses get passed on from one cell to another, thus creating a chain of information within a network of neurons.

Interestingly, nerve impulses have both an electrical and a chemical component. Electrical events trigger a signal within a neuron, and chemical processes transmit that signal from one neuron to another or to a muscle cell, to complete the circuit and produce a response.

The chemical process occurs at the end of the axon, in a structure called synapse. The axon releases chemical substances called neurotransmitters, which attach themselves to chemical receptors in the membrane of the next neuron in this complex chain, and produce excitatory or inhibitory changes (as the situation demands) in its membrane.

This is effectively the language in which brain cells "talk" to each other. When everything is in sync, the internal communications happens in such a seamless, regulated manner, that we are not at all aware of how it's happening, seemingly of its own volition.

The central nervous system communicates with the rest of the body by transmitting messages from the brain through the nerves that are connected to the spine. In addition to simple muscular activity, the CNS, as mentioned before, also controls a far more complex mind-body co-ordination by being a bridge between the chemical messenger system (CMS) and the autonomic nervous system (ANS). This complex relationship is identified as the brain neuromatrix.

CNS Functionality

The central nervous system (CNS) is the main information processing center that receives and sends information to the peripheral nervous system. The two main organs of the CNS are the brain and the spinal cord. The brain processes and interprets sensory information sent from the spinal cord. Both the brain and spinal cord have a three-layered protective, tissue covering called the meninges.

Within the CNS is a system of hollow cavities called ventricles. These cavities are filled with a cerebrospinal fluid that protects the brain and the spinal cord from all kind of trauma. It also brings nutrients to the CNS.

The Role of the Spinal Cord

The brain stem or the medulla connects the brain with the spinal cord. This part of the brain controls hunger and thirst impulses, besides regulating body temperature, blood pressure, and breathing.

The three thin membranes that cover the brain are called meninges. A watery fluid courses through four hollow spaces in the brain, called ventricles. This fluid is loaded with nutrients that it carries from the blood and delivers to the brain, while also removing the waste products from the brain.

Like the brain, the spinal cord is surrounded by cerebrospinal fluid. Spinal nerves connect the brain with other parts of the body. They transmit messages back and forth between the brain and the rest of the body.

CNS Diseases/Disorders and Treatments Available in Modern Science

The main line of treatment is drug therapy, which only gives symptomatic relief. At best, it can delay the progression of the disease, at worse it lowers the body's self-healing capacity and can even cause permanent damage.

As the CNS is the main command centre of the body, one can imagine the damage that can be caused, if this system begins to malfunction for some reason. This can turn out to be a serious issue, as despite controlling the rest of the body, the central nervous system has only a limited ability of repairing itself. A compromised CNS can also cause serious behavioural or psychological disorders.

The CNS is also vulnerable to an attack by pathogens – bacteria (bacterial meningitis), viruses (viral encephalitis), fungi (fungal meningitis, abscesses) or parasites (toxoplasmosis, cysticercosis).

Alternatively, the CNS could be affected by infections travelling from other sick organs, as in case of tuberculosis or syphilis. The meninges covering the brain system are particularly vulnerable to such infections, especially at a time a person's immunological system is weak, or compromised by pathogens.

Then there is a CNS disease called Multiple Sclerosis, that's a degenerative, autoimmune disease in which the protective covers of nerve cells of the spine or brain get severely damaged, causing serious psychiatric problems. Meningitis, arachnoid cysts and autism are other common disorders associated with CNS. CNS damage is most often permanent and non-reversible.

Severely debilitative conditions such as Dementia and Alzheimer's could be age-related progressive neurodegenerative disorders, wherein a patient gradually begins to lose all his cognitive and also motor functions.

What Causes CNS Disorders?

There could be several internal and external reasons but the most common ones are listed here:

Trauma: Depending on the site of the injury, symptoms can vary widely from paralysis to mood disorders.

Infections: some micro-organisms and viruses can invade the CNS. The most common ones are fungi, such as cryptococcal meningitis; protozoa, including malaria or bacteria, as is the case with leprosy, or viruses.

Degeneration: When the spinal cord or brain begin to gradually degenerate. A fitting example is Parkinson's disease which involves the gradual degeneration of dopamine-producing cells in the basal ganglia.

Tumours: These can be both cancerous and noncancerous tumors that can partially or wholly impair parts of the central nervous system.

Autoimmune disorders: When a person's own immune system begins to work against itself and starts attacking healthy tissues. An example is encephalomyelitis, characterized by a person's depressed immune system attacking its own myelin (the nerves' insulation) and destroying the white matter, within.

Stroke: Any blockage in the delivery of blood to the brain and the resulting lack of oxygen supply, causing premature death of the affected brain cells.

Sympathetic and Parasympathetic Nervous System

The sympathetic and parasympathetic nervous systems are the two parts of the autonomic nervous system, and are assigned an opposite set of functions. The sympathetic nervous system is in-charge of all physical and mental activity. It makes the heart beat faster and stronger, opens the airways to facilitate breathing, and inhibits digestion. In short, it's the ON switch of the body.

The parasympathetic nervous system, in contrast is the switch OFF. It's responsible for restful bodily functions. It stimulates digestion, when we are asleep; and also helps the body relax. However contrary to belief, the sympathetic and parasympathetic nervous systems do not always work at cross-purposes.

How it Works?

The parasympathetic nervous system moves along longer pathways. Preganglionic fibers from the medulla or the spinal cord project ganglia close to the target organ. They create a synapse, which eventually creates the slow response.

The sympathetic nervous system is a fast mechanism. This kind of a response is created by very short neural pathways. When a threat stimulus presents itself, it prompts the adrenal medulla to release a concoction of hormones and chemical receptors into the bloodstream, which in turn spur the various glands and muscles in the person's body. Once the perceived threat signal passes, the parasympathetic nervous system relaxes back.

Brain Dead People Are Not Actually Dead

The harshest fact of life is that death is inevitable. Yet, over the ages, we have had several well-documented cases of out-of-body and near-death experiences that have baffled scientists and left them grappling for answers. In all these reported incidents, it appears that life continues in some inexplicable manner, even after the brain has shut down completely.

A 17-year-old road accident victim, Steven Thorpe was declared brain dead by four doctors attending to him at University Hospital in Coventry, West Midlands, when his distraught parents insisted on seeking another medical opinion from their GP Julia Piper, and just moments before he was taken off the ventilator, he stirred back to life!

Scientists, across the world are confused about a clear definition of brain death. August 2016 - Nineteen days after her car flipped over, the doctors of 22-year-old Sam Hemming were about to give up on her because she was pronounced "brain dead" "with seemingly no hope of recovery". Yet moments before she was going to be unhooked from the vent, Sam wiggled her toe and left everybody aghast! Later she made a full recovery within two weeks.

January 2015 - George Pickering, a 27-year old Texan, was pronounced brain dead by doctors at the Tomball Regional Medical Center. His father was adamant he did not want his son to be taken off life support. While this face-off was happening, the son squeezed his father's hand, and went on to make a full recovery in the next few days.

March 2008 - 21-year-old Zack Dunlap was declared "brain dead" following an ATV accident. One of Zack's relatives dug a pocketknife under his fingernail, and he "woke up."

May 2008 - A Virginia family was shocked but relieved when their mother, Val Thomas, woke up after doctors declared her 'brain dead'. Doctors could read no brain waves for over 17 hours, but suddenly she woke up, as if from deep slumber and started conversing with the nurses.

In my opinion, "brain dead" doesn't mean altogether dead. Medically, a person may be declared as brain dead when their brain stem function appears to be lost.

Although brain dead humans are technically no longer alive, their bodies still circulate blood, digest food, excrete waste, and yes, even deliver a baby! Recent studies have also suggested that some electrical activity and blood flow continues after brain cell death, although it may not be enough to allow full body functioning.

We will unravel more such mysteries in our following chapters. However for this particular section, we will not consider the CNS as central nervous system + brain + spinal code but just the central nervous system, that is, only a network of nerves. Even in TCM, the meridians are independent and are not controlled by the brain. Also for this part of the book, we will consider that CNS includes the peripheral nervous system and central nervous system, but it does not include the spinal cord and the brain. In short, we will consider the entire nervous system excluding brain and spinal cord as CNS for this part of the book. And gradually, in the subsequent sections reveal the mystifying secrets about how to intelligently hack this system for healing and longevity.